"Superior stress management advice." —*Library Journal*

"Dr. Loehr has once again hit it on the head. *Toughness Training for Life* reads as a survival guide to not only my sport, tennis, but life as well." —Jim Courier, number one tennis player in the world

"Draws upon a wealth of experience in working with world-class athletes to provide a rational basis for my own personal philosophy, which is to work hard and play hard."
  —Nick Hall, Ph.D., associate professor, Department of Psychiatry
    and Behavioral Medicine, University of South Florida

"Shows us how to . . . get stronger and more productive in life . . . practical tips for people of all ages and interests."
      —Stan Smith, former number one tennis player in the world,
        U.S. Open and Wimbledon champion,
        and seven-time Davis Cup winner

"Establishes a 'mind-body connection,' which, when developed, reduces overall stress, increases energy and productivity, improves health, and helps achieve greater happiness from life."
      —*Tennis Week*

"Shows how attitude and tuning the body through exercise and diet help you deal with the ups and downs of life."
      —*Soundview Executive Book Summaries*

"Should be required reading for anyone who wants to manage stress effectively." —*Tennis* magazine

DR. JAMES E. LOEHR has trained more than 100 world-class athletes, including tennis stars Monica Seles, Pete Sampras, and Gabriela Sabatini, boxer Ray Mancini, speed skater Dan Jansen, and golfer Mark O'Mara. President and CEO of LGE Saddlebrook Sport Science Center, a research and training facility committed to teaching athletes how to attain peak performance, Loehr is the author of nine books, including *Mental Toughness Training for Sports* (Plume), *The Mental Game* (Plume), and *The New Toughness Training for Sports* (Dutton). He lives in Wesley Chapel, Florida.

JAMES E. LOEHR, Ed.D.

TOUGHNESS

TRAINING

FOR LIFE

A REVOLUTIONARY PROGRAM FOR MAXIMIZING HEALTH, HAPPINESS, AND PRODUCTIVITY

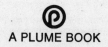

A PLUME BOOK

PLUME
Published by the Penguin Group
Penguin Books USA Inc., 375 Hudson Street, New York, New York 10014, U.S.A.
Penguin Books Ltd, 27 Wrights Lane, London W8 5TZ, England
Penguin Books Australia Ltd, Ringwood, Victoria, Australia
Penguin Books Canada Ltd, 10 Alcorn Avenue, Toronto, Ontario, Canada M4V 3B2
Penguin Books (N.Z.) Ltd, 182–190 Wairau Road, Auckland 10, New Zealand

Penguin Books Ltd, Registered Offices: Harmondsworth, Middlesex, England

Published by Plume, an imprint of Dutton Signet,
a division of Penguin Books USA Inc.
Previously published in a Dutton edition.

First Plume Printing, October, 1994
10 9 8 7 6 5

 REGISTERED TRADEMARK—MARCA REGISTRADA

The Library of Congress has catalogued the Dutton edition as follows:
Loehr, James E.
    Toughness training for life / James E. Loehr.
        p.   cm.
    Includes bibliographical references and index.
    ISBN 0-525-93612-2
    0-452-27243-2 (pbk.)
    1. Physical education and training—Psychological aspects.
    2. Physical fitness—Psychological aspects.   3. Stress management.
    I. Title.
    GV342.22.L64   1993
    796'.01—dc20   92–46914
                                                         CIP

Printed in the United States of America
Original hardcover design by Steven N. Stathakis

TO MIKE, PAT, AND JEFF
TO RENATE

ACKNOWLEDGMENTS

To Warren Jamison and Kitty Jamison for their competence and dedication in the preparation of this manuscript. To Renate Gaisser for her encouragement, technical skills, and belief. To Jack Groppel for his friendship, trust, and help. To Scott McTeer for his diligence, inspiration, and literary assistance. To Karen Elsea and Carlos Salum for their belief, vision, and support. To Peter McLaughlin for his persistence, determination, and unwavering belief. To Irv Dardik for his genius and pioneering insights into wave theory and disease reversal.

To the many people who have touched my life and made a difference with the book. To mention just a few: Tom Dempsey, Nick Hall, Paul Roetert, Pat Etcheberry, Elizabeth Backman, Tony Schwartz, Dennis Van der Meer, Laurie Williams, Dick Roberson, Ian Hamilton, Ron Woods, Joy Rodenberg, and Tim and Tom Gullikson.

CONTENTS

INTRODUCTION

Stress management systems usually aim at reducing stress, an unrealistic goal for most of us. This book shows you how to toughen up so that you can handle more stress and be healthier, happier, and more productive.

"Tough" takes on a new meaning in these pages. Not James Dean squinting over cigarette smoke, not street punks in black leather, but nice guys and gals who know how to lead happy, productive, and healthy lives.

Toughness Training for Life is a system of thinking, feeling, doing, and living that offers practical ways to solve some of life's most challenging problems. It represents a new generation of thought.

While giving you the tools to attain toughness for life, this book will answer many vital questions:

- How can I win more of life's battles, increase my productivity, and be happier and healthier?

- Why are some people mentally tough, when most are not?
- How can I become emotionally strong enough to thrive on the stress in my life?
- How can I help my kids be more persistent and resilient fighters in life's ceaseless struggles?
- What connects depression, drug abuse, and eating disorders—and how can we beat them?
- How can I make my immune system stronger?
- What can schools do to toughen children for tomorrow's more demanding world?
- How can I use emotion to maximize my productivity and performance?

As a program, Toughness Training for Life combines my clinical training and experience as a psychologist with my 16 years of sport science research and work with world-class athletes. As a book, *Toughness Training for Life* is a quantum leap from the basic model published in my earlier books *Mentally Tough* and *Mental Toughness Training for Sports*.

To say I'm excited about this program is an understatement, because it reveals so much more that we can all do to increase personal productivity, improve health, and achieve greater happiness in our lives.

Some of us have intuitively grasped elements of the program from simple truisms such as "All work and no play makes Jack a dull boy," a concept that takes on renewed meaning in these pages.

This program doesn't demand the impossible—that the stressors in our daily lives be removed. Instead it accepts life's inevitable highs and lows, its daily rhythms and oscillations, its sudden demands and constant pressures.

Toughness Training for Life is dynamically alive and excitingly challenging; it shows us how to cope head-on with life's unavoidable collisions, quarrels, and contests. Equally important, it impresses something on us that many habitually underemphasize: when and how to rest, and why rest is vital to our well-being.

Professional sports are highly visible arenas for studying stress. The physical and emotional stresses of competition break athletes in the same way that the stresses of life break people working in nonsport occupations. (By the way, "stress" is another word that we will view differently through Toughness Training for Life.)

Nowhere is the mind/body connection more evident than in competitive sport, but the lessons we learn there often have their greatest application beyond the tennis court, golf course, or playing field. They can—and should—be vital lessons for daily living.

From raising healthy, capable children to designing better educational systems, from conquering depression to breaking addiction, from raising personal performance to boosting company-wide productivity, Toughness Training for Life offers new and electrifying answers.

1

JIMMY CONNORS'S

SECRET

In the first round of the 1991 U.S. Open Tennis Tournament, 39-year-old Jimmy Connors, winner of more men's singles championships than any other player in history, is losing to the much younger Patrick McEnroe.

Between points, Connors works the crowd, shouts gibes into TV cameras, and cranks his emotional involvement in the match higher and higher. Though trailing, he fights on, his confidence unfazed, and makes one unbelievable shot after another. Patrick McEnroe, using all the youthful speed and energy at his command, responds by raising the level of his own play and fights back tenaciously. But Connors is not to be denied; at 1:35 in the morning, the veteran player nails a five-set victory.

Two rounds later, he loses the first set to 25-year-old Aaron Krickstein and trails 5–1 in the second. Connors, still cocky, still confident, still joking, wages war for every point and pulls the second set out of the fire. After losing the third, Connors wins the highly emotional fourth, and promptly falls behind 5–2 in the final set.

Krickstein, who has never lost a five-setter in the Open, now holds a commanding lead. Yet on this day he loses 7–6 in the fifth to one of the greatest fighters in the annals of sport.

Before the Open, wrist surgery sidelined Connors for a year. In spite of his abrupt drop from a 174th world ranking to as low as a dismal 990th in mid-February 1991, Jimmy has reached the semi-finals of this talent-packed grand slam event. Coaching wisdom holds that old guys don't come back in tennis, yet wise coaches also know that Connors is no ordinary player.

Like 20,000 others packing the stadium, I sit on the edge of my seat waiting to see if the aging miracle man of tennis will do it again in the semifinals. Jimmy seizes his moments of glory, pumping both hands in the air to celebrate return-of-serve winners. However, his opponent this day is another player of unshakable confidence, Jim Courier, the 21-year-old in a baseball cap soon to be ranked number one in the world. Connors loses, but his battle against all odds is a gripping comeback story.

Not as strong, quick, or agile as many of his youthful compet-itors, Jimmy clearly knows how to rise above physical limitations and perform magnificently under pressure. Just as clearly, the sig-nificance of his competitive spirit extends far beyond the limited scope of professional sport.

What's his secret? Is it just a peculiar thing, unique to Jimmy Connors and a few other sports champions, or is it a set of univer-sal principles that can be learned by anyone and applied to every aspect of life?

I've spent a good part of my professional career trying to grasp what makes great competitors like Jimmy Connors so tough. I've discovered that understanding their distinctive response to stress and their uncanny ability to transcend the impairments of pressure is important to everyone. Jimmy Connors, the super-performer and mega-competitor, is mentally one of the toughest athletes of all time. What Connors and others like him do holds great promise for us all.

Nothing displays a person's toughness more than her or his per-formance when the stakes are highest. In this regard, contrasting

Connors with his less accomplished competitors provides many fundamental insights. When he is at his best, Connors's response is passionate high energy; theirs often is withdrawn, quiet, nonengaging. The force of his will is intimidating; his determination to fight through to victory rises like a powerful storm. Connors's walk and posture under fire communicates strength, purpose, and confidence. No dragging, no stooped shoulders. At his top form, Connors's positive self-talk leaves no room in his mind to review negative developments or entertain self-defeating thoughts.

Perhaps Connors's greatest competitive attribute is his capacity to carve out a sense of fun and joy as the battle rages. His love for the game and competition is so powerfully communicated that his fans become infected with the same passion and excitement.

It's clear that mentally tough athletes like Connors have developed a capacity for a remarkable emotional response under stress, a response that precisely defines their genius as competitors. The biochemistry driven by this special emotional response delivers extraordinary powers to the physical body. Hands, eyes, and feet shift into perfectly coordinated hypergear; talent, skill, and desire blend effortlessly to deliver amazing performances.

THE TOUGHNESS RESPONSE THAT WINS

Exactly what is this remarkable emotional impulse, this biochemically driven response that defines the successful competitor in any field?

I call it the Toughness Response. It rises from four distinct response capacities:

1. Emotional Flexibility
Emotional flexibility is the capacity to remain open and nondefensive in the highly stressed competitive situations of living, whether one meets them in business, sport, or personal life. People who have developed emotional flexibility can summon a wide range of positive emotions (humor, joy, fun, fighting spirit, etc.) without regard to competitive conditions or outcomes. This flexibility brings perspective and emotional balance, thereby preserving one's creativity and problem-solving ability.

2. Emotional Responsiveness

When they compete, the emotionally tough are fully alive emotionally to the present; they are not locked up, withdrawn, or mentally absent. They are able to be themselves in the most positive and constructive way. Their emotional responsiveness keeps them alert, tuned-in, and fully engaged in the competitive struggle at hand.

3. Emotional Strength

Under pressure, the mentally tough are passionate. By generating great emotion they are able to resist intense force from their competition. This capacity—the ability to summon high levels of positive emotional strength under the most stressful circumstances—is the trademark of the consummate competitor.

4. Emotional Resiliency

One learns most about an athlete's mental toughness by observing how quickly he or she bounces back from emotional hits—missing free throws, double-faulting on break points, fumbling a touchdown pass. Watch the truly great competitors when they're losing or playing badly. They can take an emotional hit—lots of hits—and be right back in your face, hammering at your weak points, forcing you to make mistakes.

The capacity to bounce back emotionally is a critical part of mental toughness.

―――――――――― **MENTAL TOUGHNESS IN YOUR LIFE** ――――――――――

From the outside, the world of big-time sport seems glamorous, an enchanted place where dreams come true. On the inside, the work is demanding and repetitive, the competition fierce and unrelenting, the pressures complex and constant. Once the psychological reality of sport is understood, establishing the importance of mental toughness is easy. But this is a book about life, not merely sport. How important is mental toughness in life? What is the psychological reality of stress in our personal lives?

Despite all our technological progress, life today is emotionally demanding and surprisingly stressful. This is true for single working mothers, corporation presidents, and everyone else who must juggle the conflicting demands of work, family, health, finances, and myriad other concerns—in other words, just about everybody.

IS CLAUDIA BROOKS'S STORY LIKE YOURS?

A glimpse into two versions of a day in the life of Claudia Brooks can give us a quick understanding of the vast difference between nontough and tough responses in the nonsport world.

Claudia is 37, the divorced mother of two children, ages 5 and 9. She works for a small computer software company as a sales representative. All across America, millions of Claudias struggle to survive.

A typical day for Claudia:

Up at 6:15, prepare breakfast. Sharon to preschool and Andy to elementary school by 7:45. Today is important because she meets with the bank to discuss her delinquent house and car payments; one of her major worries at the moment is that the bank will force the sale of her home. Claudia's ex-husband consistently fails to make his child support and alimony payments, and, in a market hit hard by recession, her take-home pay has dropped significantly during the past eight months.

Claudia has other worries. Rumor has it that her employer, Benson Software, is also in serious financial trouble. Two other sales reps were laid off last month, and Claudia's greatest fear has been that she might be next. Her savings are gone and her parents are barely scraping by. The bills continue to pile up; her car has passed the 100,000-mile mark and requires major repairs, and she learned yesterday that her 5-year-old needs extensive dental work to correct a serious overbite.

This afternoon Claudia has two sales appointments that could help her financial situation tremendously. The appointments are scheduled just before her late-afternoon bank meeting. She knows that if she lets her emotions get in the way, she'll never be able to close the sales. And tonight is Andy's birthday party. No matter what happens at the bank, she doesn't want to ruin his birthday. She would never forgive herself.

Claudia's day of balancing financial strains, job insecurity, sales pressure, and parenting responsibilities is a standard day for millions of people. Claudia's financial options are closing, but the real issue is her performance. Can she manage her emotions? Can she still sell? Can she think clearly? Can Claudia tough it out—and pound out workable solutions? If she can bring all her talent and skill to the table, if she can perform superbly in her sales calls and with the bank manager, her chances are good.

The following two scenarios contrast how a nontough Claudia might handle this stress overload compared to how a toughened Claudia would respond.

CLAUDIA'S NONTOUGH RESPONSE

It's never been this bad, Claudia thinks, anxiously glancing at her watch. Why do I have to be stuck in traffic today of all days?

Gripping the steering wheel like a life preserver, she stares blankly ahead, her mind too far away to notice that her lane must merge to the left. A loud horn reminds her that she must yield; she slams on her brakes just in time to avoid a large Mercedes. Glancing over, she catches the lady's reproachful look.

Heart racing, Claudia's face sours as she watches the sleek car glide past. With a quick motion she jerks her car into the proper lane, silently cursing whoever is responsible for not marking the road better. As she joins the regular flow of traffic, her car's engine groans and sputters, reminding her again of her impossible financial situation. She feels miserable enough to pull over and have a good cry.

At the office things don't seem much better. The recent layoffs mean there's more work to do, and she's the one who has to do it. Obviously this morning is no exception. Today's paperwork will take the entire morning.

She has other things to do: prepare for this afternoon's sales meetings and schedule more appointments for the rest of the week. She spends a few moments grousing to herself about the ridiculously low salary Benson Software pays; sales commissions are the only decent money she makes.

"How in hell am I going to get rid of this junk in time to do myself some good?" Claudia mutters as she leafs through the papers. She knows she has to pull herself together to face the bank manager; her fate is in his hands. Wishing she were anywhere but here, Claudia stares at the papers in front of her as though they were ancient Latin scrolls, her mind heavy. At last she slowly begins to dispose of the paperwork, her thoughts struggling through the glue of her personal problems.

She arrives at her first sales appointment promptly. Claudia gives the secretary her name, but the small lady seems confused.

"Was Mr. Phillips expecting you?"

"Yes, at two o'clock. I have an appointment."

"I don't have you down here. Did you speak to . . . ?"

"I spoke to Mr. Phillips. 'Two o'clock Monday' were his exact words."

"I'm sorry, Ms. Brooks, but he doesn't have it in his appointment book, and . . ."

"Is he here?"

"He went out to our valley plant this morning. I don't expect him back today. But I can . . ."

"Just tell him I was here and he wasn't. Here's my card; he can call me if he likes."

The secretary conceals her annoyance. "I'll certainly give him the message, Ms. Brooks."

Claudia storms out, so possessed by rage that she talks to herself. "What did I do to deserve all this hassle? What a nightmare day."

With her next appointment scheduled for 3:00, Claudia drives to a nearby fast-food restaurant. She didn't make time for breakfast, and now she's not only furious but weak with hunger. She thinks aloud, "Maybe some quick food will help."

Eating gives her something to do, a diversion of sorts. Nevertheless, as usual when she's nervous or angry, Claudia finds it almost impossible to get food down. Suddenly she feels alarmingly tired, and wishes she could take a long nap.

But she can't nap. Gotta go, gotta go, she chants to herself as she realizes that her spare hour is slipping away, her next meeting is on the other side of town, and she isn't sure how to get there.

After a stressful rush across town, Claudia at last is sitting across the desk from the dynamic vice president of a rapidly growing company. "So what can you do for us?" the man asks.

To answer this simple and direct question, Claudia struggles to organize an effective response. Her thoughts are shaky and disjointed, her words scrambled.

"Ms. Brooks, what do you know about our company?"

"Well, ah . . ."

"Do you even know what we do here?"

Claudia does, but for the moment a coherent answer seems light years away. Her eyes fall to the floor. Why are you being so aggressive with me? she thinks, knowing she's choking, that she's blowing the opportunity.

Pulling into the bank's parking lot a little later, Claudia feels overwhelmed. On top of all her other burdens, she can't put the embarrassing disaster of the day's only sales call out of her mind. She walks toward the bank, her shoulders drooping, her step tentative, aware that her life is spinning out of control. She has only one hope now: that someone will have sympathy for her situation. Maybe one person will at least show a little compassion and sensitivity. Maybe things will somehow work out after all. Maybe, maybe, maybe . . .

CLAUDIA'S TOUGH RESPONSE

With the kids safely stowed away at school, Claudia moves onto the freeway. A few miles down the road she enters the jam, taking her place behind a long line of cars creeping along. "Maybe an accident," she mutters.

No problem, she thinks, refusing to let anything complicate her situation further. Not today. Humming softly to herself, Claudia pops a cassette into the tape deck. Sitting up straight, she takes a deep breath and feels her body settle into the seat.

With this much traffic there'll be more time for music, more time to get myself together, Claudia tells herself. Today I definitely need it.

Listening to the soothing notes pouring out of the rear speakers, Claudia decides the traffic delay is a blessing in disguise.

A couple of hundred yards ahead she sees a merge sign. Flipping her blinker on, Claudia glances to her left and puts on her "May I?" expression.

A lady in a large Mercedes returns Claudia's smile with an "After you" gesture. Claudia waves back, gives the accelerator a light

punch, and waits while the engine decides whether to accept the order. A half-second later her car lurches forward with a groan.

"Hang in there," she says, patting the dashboard as if the car
were a sick child. "We'll make it." Suddenly her eyes fill with tears
as the reality of her situation hits her again. "Not now," she says
out loud, reaching down to turn Beethoven up a few notches. "Not
now!"

At work there is much to be done. Anticipating the shortness
of time and her inability to eat when nervous or upset, she has
packed juice and her favorite liquid meal. This gives her a few extra
minutes to prepare for her sales appointments. Claudia knew the
night before that she'd need the extra time.

The recession has been difficult for Benson Software Corporation. Good people, livewood people, laid off; vital projects stretched
out; new products delayed. Under such circumstances, Claudia
knows that only the most valuable and productive will keep their
jobs. Fortunately her boss has confidence in her despite a recent
lack of sales; he is giving Claudia more time to demonstrate her
skills.

Claudia reviews her notes on the day's prospective clients,
pausing every so often to breathe deeply and assure herself that
she will be okay. In quick bursts, connections are made. If ever
there was a company in need of what Benson Software provides,
Phillips Industries is it. "Like a hand and a glove," she whispers ex-
citedly to herself, snapping her briefcase shut. "Let's go do it!"

"He's not in, Ms. Brooks. Was Mr. Phillips expecting you?"

"I thought so, but maybe we were supposed to touch base
again first."

The small lady peers up from her desk at the young woman.
She likes Claudia's style and easy manner. Obviously, Mr. Phillips
has forgotten another appointment. Again she will cover for her
busy boss, but today it won't be hard. The person in front of her
isn't trying to make matters worse.

"I'll tell Mr. Phillips you dropped by, and see if I can get the
two of you together tomorrow to talk business."

Claudia smiles appreciatively, her face still strong and confident. She feels sure that things will work out on this sale. "Thanks.
Just tell Mr. Phillips that I can save his company a lot of money."

The secretary's face lights up with a pleasant smile. "I'm sure you can. Don't worry, I'll have Mr. Phillips call you first thing in the morning. By the way, my name's Dolly."

"Thanks, Dolly." Claudia's smile is genuine. The no-show means she has time to grab a few things for Andy's party.

After buying balloons, water pistols, and hats, Claudia still has twenty extra minutes to review her notes for the 3:00 appointment.

"What can Benson Software do for us?" the vice president's strong voice fires out.

With a confident smile Claudia says, "I was hoping you'd ask that."

At the bank, Claudia needs no sympathy. She is composed, her mind lucid. With confident excitement she reports that her second sales call looks very promising for a large commission, and on the first she had high hopes of making another lucrative sale.

"Two big hits in one day—this is the turning point I've been looking for." Claudia asks for forty-five days to bring her payments current—and gets it.

Driving home, tears of relief roll down Claudia's cheeks. "I did it, I did it. And tomorrow I'll do it again!" But tonight her son would be the happiest 9-year-old in the state. "That's a promise," she says to herself. "That's a promise."

YOUR PERFORMANCE UNDER PRESSURE

At first glance you may have trouble seeing the connection between Jimmy Connors's age problems, Claudia's financial problems, and your life. If so, let's connect Connors and Claudia first, and then show how the tough response relates to your life.

Connors has everything to gain; Claudia has everything to lose. He has the crowds on his side; she has no one. He's doing what he loves; she's doing what she must.

Taking the comparison further reveals significant points. Both Connors and Claudia are fighting huge personal battles. For both, the stakes are high, the performance challenges formidable.

For Connors, winning demands total concentration, clear thinking, and precise execution of ground strokes, serves, passing shots, and playing tactics—under pressure. For Claudia, winning demands nearly identical concentration, clear thinking, and precise execution of her duties, responsibilities, and selling tactics—under pressure. Only the mechanical requirements in each arena are different—running, jumping, and hitting versus communicating, negotiating, and closing. The essential emotional requirements are identical.

The emotional requirements you face in winning against the challenges, stresses, and opportunities in your life are universal. So are mine. So are every businessperson's, every college student's, every employee's. In other words, your emotional requirements are identical to those faced by Connors and Claudia.

THE ESSENCE OF TOUGHNESS— KNOWING HOW TO TURN YOUR IPS ON

Tough Claudia sailed through her performance day by being emotionally flexible, responsive, strong, and resilient. This enabled her to tap into her Ideal Performance State (IPS). She fought the day's battles, enjoyed the day's challenges, and savored the day's successes much as any professional athlete might in baseball, skiing, or beach volleyball.

Years of work with struggling athletes has taught me that success in sport is linked more to one's ability to control this special emotional condition, the IPS, than to talent or skill. IPS control brings balance, perspective, enjoyment, poise, calmness, positive energy, and passion to the battle.

The discovery that fulfillment of athletic potential and IPS control are inseparably linked was a great breakthrough. Put simply, when a person's emotional condition is right, he or she performs right.

That the IPS exists has been proved repeatedly by athletes who speak of playing "in the zone," of "treeing," of perceiving a tennis ball to be "as big as a giant grapefruit." Some comedians, writers, and salespeople think of IPS as being "on a roll"; others call it "grooving." Everyone experiencing the IPS seems to have the same feeling: that nothing can go wrong, that play or performance just flows and success is assured.

Awareness of the existence of the IPS led to a perplexing challenge. How could the IPS and the Toughness Response be measured, identified, and harnessed for the benefit of everyone if we can't even see it?

Sometimes things most real are those we can't see. I recall what the fox told the little prince in Antoine de Saint Exupéry's classic:

> ... here is my secret, a very simple secret: it is only with the heart that one can see rightly; what is essential is invisible to the eye. "What is essential is invisible to the eye," the little prince repeated, so he would be sure to remember.

How could we unlock the secret of the IPS, the secret athletes speak of so convincingly, the secret state the best of them can tap into at will? The possibilities of solving this challenge were tremendously exciting. Why couldn't athletes who had never experienced the IPS also learn to tap into it? And why couldn't the same principles be applied to life in general?

THE TOUGHNESS LINK TO LIFE

The link between success in life and the mental toughness that makes it possible to reach one's IPS—whether that success be in business, parenting, or achievement in any other field—became apparent rather quickly. Exactly how we achieve this mental state, this mental toughness, was the mystery and the continuing stimulus for my research into this invisible world. Seeing the relationship of IPS to physical nature only sweetened the search. Indeed, the exact nature of the mental toughening process—the way IPS control is learned—remained incomplete and inadequate until quite recently.

Intuitively, I knew the toughening process is linked to cycles of stress and recovery in some tangible way; exactly how and why began to unfold late in 1990. During a period of intense work and study from 1989 to 1991, partial answers began to emerge from research in developmental and clinical psychology as well as sport psychology, and from a wide diversity of interdisciplinary sciences—exercise physiology, chronobiology, psychoneuroimmun-ology, and biochemistry.

My clients made dramatic improvements during this period, al-most entirely because of this new understanding and approach to training. Tennis players Gabriela Sabatini, Shuzo Matsuoka, David Wheaton, and Sergi Bruguera, Olympic speed skaters Dan Jansen and Nick Thometz, and scores of others experienced quantum leaps in performance.

For the first time in my professional career, I have a working understanding of how stress affects us, both physically and emo-tionally; how it strengthens us and how it weakens us. More impor-tant, I now understand how this knowledge can be harnessed to improve our daily lives.

IPS control in sport demands great toughness—meaning the ability to act with flexibility, responsiveness, strength, and resili-ency. Paralleling sport, if we are to lead highly productive, happy, and healthy lives, we must also learn to reach our IPS by develop-ing our toughness. I'm excited because the tools are now here—in these pages—to make toughness an attainable life skill for every-one.

SUMMARY

Emotion rules sport and life. Passion, joy, love, confidence, hope, and even happiness are feelings and emotions. The right emotions empower our physical bodies and free our spirits. The wrong emo-tions block, trap, and blind us. Fear, anger, fatigue, and uncon-trolled depression disempower us—often to a tragic degree—by setting up panic, mistakes, accidents, failures, poor health, and un-happiness. Clearly, toughness is vital to athletes; it is equally impor-tant to all of us.

Maximum productivity, health, and happiness are universal goals. That's what toughness promises—and delivers. Lacking toughness, you have to settle for less than your maximum potential, often for much, much less.

This book is based on my belief in these premises:

- Toughness is both emotional and physical.
- Toughness is flexibility, responsiveness, strength, and resiliency under stress.
- In life, as in sport, the emotions rule.
- Toughness Training puts you in control of your performance level in your career and in your private life.
- Achieving maximum productivity, health, and happiness demands toughness.

2

HOW YOU

CAN GET

TOUGH

Get tough. Tough it out. Save your business and beat the competition with tough-minded management. Have you ever been prodded by this kind of advice?

Jimmy Connors and Claudia know how to tough it out. In pressure-filled situations they respond with great toughness. Because they are able to display the four core elements of mental and emotional health—flexibility, responsiveness, strength, and resiliency—they can function in their Ideal Performance States and achieve their maximum potential. We can say they are mentally tough.

The four core qualities are not limited to emotional or mental toughness. They are also characteristic of a healthy physical body and can even be observed in nature.

Do you recall Aesop's Fable of the oak and willow? The proud and rigid oak boasted of his strength to his neighbor, the delicate and sensitive willow. Even the slightest breeze caused her to sway and bend, while the oak stood like a granite cliff.

Eventually a greater wind than had ever swept across the country struck the oak's rigid trunk, splintering it. The oak lost many large branches before the great wind died away, leaving only a shattered skeleton of the huge tree. Yet the willow—flexible, responsive, and resilient—came through unharmed, still strong and undamaged despite being buffeted by gusting, swirling forces.

We may not be emotionally or physically flexible, responsive, strong, and resilient now, but we can acquire the ability to respond in this manner. The critical issue is how.

In my evolving study of mental toughness, I examined the emotional toughening process by tackling the precise process of physical toughening. Healthy, toughened muscles, cardiovascular systems, and immune systems, I discovered, possess the same response capabilities as healthy emotions.

What exciting and encouraging news! We were on the right track. The suspected links did exist. This meant that health is health, whether physical or emotional. In addition, I realized that toughness, as I had come to use the term, is health at a very high level. This is the fundamental element of Toughness Training for Life.

HOW TOUGHNESS TRAINING FOR LIFE IS DIFFERENT

Toughness Training departs from traditional stress management models in many ways. In particular it follows natural laws and is based on measurable scientific data; therefore it is both logical and practical. More to the point—it works.

In traditional stress models, the central focus is on stress management; the ultimate goal is complete freedom from emotional stress. Great idea. Easier said than done in today's hectic world, where we have little control over many factors that assault us. The wind that broke the oak but only swayed the willow, the obstacles and frustrations that Claudia encounters in her workday, the field of strong young competitors eager to defeat Connors—all are much like the challenges life throws at you.

Current stress management strategies invariably advocate one

of two methods of controlling stress: remove the stressors altogether, or reduce one's emotional response to them. The idea has
been that if you can't handle the volume of stress in your life and
you can't remove the stressors, then the only real alternative is to
harden yourself—to become less responsive and less sensitive to
the world around you.

In the context of the Toughness Training model, toughness
and health are defined in terms of:

1. An increased capacity to expend energy—that is, to sustain a
   greater volume of stress both physically and emotionally;
2. An increased capacity to recover energy—that is, to sustain a
   greater volume of recovery both physically and emotionally.

The dominant theme of the traditional strategies has been protection from stress. Within that context, to quiet, to subdue, to become
linear is to move in the direction of control and health. In these traditional models, effective stress management is movement toward
homeostasis and equilibrium. Little or no attention is paid to the
process that permits individuals to get stronger and expand their
capacity to cope with stress. Yet if we observe our world and our
bodies, we must conclude that all life is dynamic and that the static
model goes against nature.

Life flows in ups and downs; it is not homeostatic. The healthy
heart on an EKG machine shows rhythmic peaks and valleys; a flat
line means death—the ultimate linearity. In vivid contrast, spikes
mean energy, arousal, action—life.

The same is true of our measurements of brain waves. Equilibrium is achieved through a balance of peaks and valleys, not
through living a linear existence. Further proof of this contention
lies in the circadian rhythms of our bodies, the ebb and flow of the
tides, the seasonal cycles when nature recovers energy in the fall
and winter after expending great energy in the spring and summer.

THE BASIS OF
TOUGHNESS TRAINING FOR LIFE

As your coach, I want you to get specially prepared for this section of the chapter. It's going to be a little tough to read—somewhat like a textbook filled with definitions. All these terms have special meanings in Toughness Training. Absorb what you can on the first reading and that's all you'll need. For easy reference, the terms are also listed alphabetically in a glossary at the end of the book.

The Toughness Training for Life model is based on the following basic definitions and concepts.

───────────────── **DEFINITIONS** ─────────────────

- **The Ideal Performance State (IPS)** is the most effective and reliable mental, emotional, and physical state for performing at one's best. IPS is characterized by a specific constellation of positive feelings and emotions—calmness, relaxation, confidence, joy, and a sense of fun and fulfillment.
- **IPS Control** is the ability to put oneself into the Ideal Performance State whenever desired in order to function at one's highest level. This priceless skill is acquired through Toughness Training.
- **Health** is action, movement, oscillation, and pulsation. Nonlinearity, both physically and emotionally, is the goal. When this goal is approached, the dynamic interactions of stress and recovery are in balance; this balance brings psychological and physical harmony and synchrony.
- **Healthiness,** to go a step further, is the direct consequence of regular, repeated cycles of balanced stress and recovery. Protection from stress breeds linearity, which in any form eventually becomes dysfunctional and unhealthy. Toughness is dynamic, not static; fluctuating, not stationary. Its measure is flexibility, responsiveness, strength, and resiliency under stress.
- **Stress** means anything that causes energy to be expended; recovery is anything that causes energy to be recaptured. Both stress and recovery are biochemical events. Mental and emotional stress is just as real and tangible as that of the physical

body because energy expenditure occurs physically, mentally, and emotionally. We can experience two kinds of stress:

1. *Positive stress.* Energy expenditure without physical or emotional pain is positive stress, the kind most likely to toughen you.
2. *Negative stress.* Energy expenditure accompanied by physical or emotional pain is negative stress, and is the kind most likely to weaken you.

- **Positive emotions** include joy, love, pleasure, laughter, confidence, fighting spirit, celebration of victory, warmth, and security.
- **Negative emotions** include guilt, anger, and fear—the language of psychological pain. They are critical barometers of excessive, linear stress.
- **Pain,** physical or emotional, is a signal to stop. Discomfort is a signal to pay attention.
- **To toughen** is to become more flexible, responsive, strong, and resilient—emotionally, mentally, or physically—in response to stress.
- **To weaken** is to become less flexible, responsive, energetic, and resilient—either physically or emotionally—in response to stress.
- **Weakened individuals** respond to stress in rigid, defensive, non-adaptive ways, particularly in business and other nonsport situations. Their slow and indecisive responses often lack energy and force. In addition, weakened individuals show a distinct inability to recover quickly from episodes of stress.
- **Toughness Training,** which may be either physical or emotional, exposes a weakened individual to positive challenges of sufficient intensity to cause adaptation to a higher level of stress. Toughening results from the systematic and precise administration of cycles of energy expenditure (stress) alternating with properly balanced cycles of energy recovery (rest). No stress means no toughening; excessive stress also means no toughening. In contrast, balancing the proper level of stress for a given individual with adequate recovery causes toughening.
- **Challenges** are opportunities to go beyond one's normal limits by sustaining greater than usual stress. If challenges are part of

a consistent program, accepting them enables one to reach higher levels of adaptation and toughness.

- **Overtraining** results when more stress than recovery is sought (or endured) over an extended period of time. Flexibility, responsiveness, strength, and resiliency all decline in overtraining, resulting in weakening.
- **Undertraining** occurs when one has more recovery than stress over an extended period of time. This absence of challenge weakens the overly rested individual.
- **Stress management** is the art and science of balancing the nearly endless symphony of pulsating stress and recovery clocks that influence all human beings.
- **Linearity** is being in a rut—rigidly adhering to routines and activities that provide little variation in the levels of activity and stress, which may be constantly high or constantly low. Linearity (a term coined by Irv Dardik) is the opposite of the oscillating cycles of stress and recovery that characterize action, movement, and toughening.

PUTTING TOUGHNESS TRAINING TO WORK IN YOUR DAILY LIFE

Understanding how I arrived at these definitions will help you put the model to work in your daily life. Once you become comfortable with the basic findings that support the Toughness Training for Life model, you will have a firm grasp on the similarities and interrelationships between emotional, mental, and physical health. The more thorough your understanding, the easier it will be to use mental toughness to attain your Ideal Performance State.

With these Toughness Training for Life precepts in mind, let's more closely examine health and its four attributes: flexibility, responsiveness, strength, and resiliency.

HEALTHY MUSCLES

What differentiates healthy muscles from unhealthy ones?

First, a healthy muscle remains *flexible* when stressed. This means that against resistance it is capable of a full range of motion without pain. In contrast, an inflexible muscle is unhealthy, since it does not adapt well to sudden changes in force, resistance, and direction. Also, it's more prone to injury and breakdown.

Because inflexible muscles are incapable of bending much in response to stress, they are easily extended beyond their effective range of coping. What is true of muscles is also true of the entire person: Inflexible people are easily extended beyond their effective range of coping—often with unfortunate to disastrous results. Whether emotionally or physically, the capacity to respond with flexibility is an indication of health.

A healthy muscle responds to stimulation, even subtle stimulation. The quicker and more sensitive the muscle, the healthier it is. In contrast, slow, nonresponsive muscles are unhealthy, much like the complete person who possesses such muscles. Nonresponsive muscles or people are nonadaptive, insensitive, and potentially dysfunctional. On the other hand, healthy people are *responsive*.

A healthy muscle is also *strong*. In the physical world, toughening means strengthening—increasing the capacity to generate and expend energy. Both toughened muscles and toughened people are capable of generating and resisting great amounts of energy and force.

And finally, a healthy muscle is *resilient;* it recovers quickly from stress. In fact, one of the best indicators of muscular (as well as cardiovascular) fitness is recovery time. A speedy, complete recovery indicates a high level of health and fitness, hence toughness. A sluggish, partial recovery, on the other hand, is a sign of nonhealth. Slow recovery from physical stress reveals insufficient physical toughness, just as slow recovery from emotional stress reveals insufficient emotional toughness.

HEALTHY MIND

Given the striking parallels between physical and emotional toughness, I was hopeful that probing deeper into the exact nature of the physical toughening process would lead to important insights into emotional toughening. My hunch was that understanding flexibility, responsiveness, strength, and resiliency in physical training would prove helpful to developing a better understanding of how emotional toughness is acquired. My further research, experimentation, and analysis established that such is most definitely the case.

From the beginning it was clear that toughening the muscles and the body would be easier to monitor than toughening the emotions and the mind. So to make it easier for you to grasp how the Toughness Training for Life model can work in your life, we'll begin with muscles.

HOW TO MAXIMIZE
THE EFFICIENCY OF YOUR
PHYSICAL TOUGHENING PROGRAM

Striking the proper balance between stress and recovery is a crucial but often undervalued consideration in physical training. Generally, specific exercises are done that are designed to gradually stretch or strengthen a muscle (or increase its flexibility, responsiveness, and resiliency) over time. While a given muscle is progressively challenged beyond its normal limits, an adaptation occurs in the muscle that allows it to extend beyond its previous level of toughness. "Training effect" is a direct result of the training stress, whether in the area of flexibility, responsiveness, strength, or resiliency. The similarities are clear.

TRAINING MUSCLE STRENGTH

You're an avid skier. Feeling unusually brave one morning, you decide to really challenge the slopes. Rocketing down the mountain, you prejump the moguls with perfect timing. All goes well until you suddenly ski onto a patch of blue ice, lose control, and thump into a solid snowbank at high speed.

Slowly your eyes open. For a moment you think you've escaped injury, although your right arm is numb below the elbow. But when you start to get up, sharp pain lets you know you're not getting off easy. In the emergency room an hour later, X-rays eliminate any lingering hope: Your right forearm's radius (large bone) is badly fractured, and you'll be in a cast for two months.

Two months of doing everything left-handed pass slowly until at last the moment arrives to remove the cast. When the doctor takes it off you gasp at the sight. Can that withered limb really be your arm?

The Effect of No Stress at All

What you see is a muscle group that has been completely protected from stress. As you move your arm around, it becomes painfully obvious that the size, responsiveness, coordination, and strength of your forearm has been dramatically reduced. This extreme example illustrates that in our context of toughening, completely protecting muscles from stress weakens rather than toughens the muscles involved.

Rehabilitation

At this point your orthopedic surgeon strongly urges you to go through the rehabilitation process. Naturally you agree and eagerly begin therapy. Heeding your doctor's advice, you take it very easy for a few weeks. Although you are careful not to overstress your arm, you do stimulate (exercise) the muscles—challenge them—more than when your arm was completely immobilized. In addition, you follow the doctor's orders and give the muscles periods of complete rest by placing your arm in a sling at regular intervals. To your great relief, the toughening process takes place before your eyes.

From this we see that even a severely weakened muscle can be toughened by exposure to intermittent, progressively increasing cycles of mild stress without pain. These cycles of stress must alternate with regular periods of rest and recovery.

BUILDING PHYSICAL POWER

The process whereby muscles are weakened and strengthened is becoming clear, but taking our analogy one step further will tell us even more. Exactly six months after your accident your doctor gives you a final checkup. Completely satisfied with your progress, he gives you permission to resume all your activities. Although your arm is within 10 percent of its full strength and coordination, you want to continue your strength-building program. You want to look, feel, and be stronger.

To increase the strength of your arm, several factors must be considered. The first is that maintaining the current level of stress on your arm will not cause strength increases. Strength gains occur only when the muscles are stressed (loaded) beyond the point where they are normally stressed. This is called the overload principle.

The second important factor is that while muscles must be stressed against a proportionately greater level of resistance to become stronger, overstresses must be avoided. If the level of resistance is too great for current capacities, the muscles being overstressed may actually lose, rather than gain, strength. In addition, the risk of injury in overstressing is quite high.

TRAINING MUSCLE FLEXIBILITY

We increase the flexibility of a particular muscle when we expand the range of motion through which it can move without pain. Again, flexibility will increase only when periods of recovery (relaxation/nonstretching) balance the doses of stress (contraction/stretching).

How hard we push ourselves—the intensity and duration of the stress—and the duration of the period between stress determine whether we are toughening the muscle effectively.

Excessive stretching with insufficient recovery relative to stress simply surpasses the adaptive capacity of the muscle and is generally accompanied by pain. So throw out the popular adage "No pain, no gain," an idea that does more harm than good.

The no-pain-no-gain myth is merely counterproductive if not pushed too far. However, if you have a high pain threshold, practicing no-pain-no-gain can stiffen you up severely and even do permanent damage to ligaments and joints. Keep in mind that physical pain is the body's way of telling you the training stress is too demanding, and that you're risking muscular injury or breakdown if you don't ease back.

Contrast overstretching with inadequate recovery time to insufficient stretching with too much recovery in relation to the stress imposed. Since the training stress is not significant in the second case, no adaptation will occur. In other words, nothing happens. Again we look for balance. As we will learn in much more detail later, the key factor in achieving the desired adaptation (increase in flexibility) is exposure to properly balanced and controlled cycles of stress and recovery without pain.

TRAINING MUSCLE RESPONSIVENESS

A healthy muscle is responsive. To be tough, it must be highly responsive.

The complex attribute of muscle responsiveness is determined by a number of interrelated factors. Among these are motor-neuron and muscle-fiber healthiness, nerve-impulse sensitivity, neuron diameter, muscle-fiber type, receptor-site responsiveness, neural-drive level, and synchronization of motor-unit firing.

Exercising muscles causes specific changes in the hormones being released from the endocrine system, which helps the muscles make their toughening adaptation. Thus, when muscles are stressed and stimulated, chemical messengers are released into the bloodstream. Although these chemical messengers are primarily targeted for specific tissue cells, nearly every physiological function of the body is affected by their release. During muscle exercise, the neuroendocrine connection is also stimulated, which also contributes to the muscle's overall responsiveness.

Research shows that regular doses of planned exercise have positive effects on all the variables that affect muscle responsiveness. "Use it or lose it" applies here. Like increasing flexibility and strength, increasing muscle responsiveness requires the proper level of increased stimulation. Excessive stimulation can weaken muscles, causing them to be less responsive and sensitive to challenges, less effective in performance.

Thus, when muscles are properly trained through balanced cycles of appropriate stress and recovery, a variety of physiological and biochemical adaptations occur that lead to improved responsiveness. However, when the same muscles are overtrained or undertrained, the desired adaptations do not take place.

TRAINING MUSCLE RESILIENCY

A well-trained, toughened muscle recovers from periods of stress much faster than an untrained muscle. In fact, measuring the heart's recovery speed after stress is one of the most widely used measures for assessing an individual's health and fitness.

Like any muscle, the cardiovascular system (lungs and heart) requires exercise in order to increase recovery speed. Increases in resiliency are determined by the volume, frequency, duration, and intensity of training stress, as well as the timing and duration of recovery.

Properly designed cycles of stress (exercise), whether aerobic or anaerobic, result in improved muscular recovery and resiliency because of the physiological and biochemical adaptations that occur. In one of the more important adaptations that result, the capillaries surrounding each muscle increase in number. This adaptation occurs because greater stress causes an increased exchange of fuels and gases between the blood and the muscle; this forces the body to form more capillaries, which generate faster recovery and greater resiliency. Additional adaptations include a larger and more efficient oxygen delivery system, as well as increased red blood cell volume. These adaptations are part of the overall toughening of the muscle.

Toughening Process Adaptations Are Real and Measurable

It's not vital that you take time to learn how and why these adaptations take place; it's more important to know that the adaptations involved in the toughening process are real and measurable. For our purposes the most important understanding is that these adaptations, which require time, will not occur if the cycles of stress and recovery are either excessive (overtraining) or insufficient (undertraining).

--- EMOTIONAL TOUGHENING ---

Gaining an understanding of the roles played by flexibility, responsiveness, strength, and resiliency in physical toughening drove me onward. It spurred my hope that the principles of adaptation would apply to emotional toughening as well. The greatest challenge came in trying to grasp where mental toughness adaptations take place. Although it was clear that physical toughening produced measurable physical adaptations, one important question remained: What adaptations occur in emotional toughening? If these emotional changes were real, it seemed logical that there would be measurable corresponding adaptations.

When the Chemistry Is Right

Intuitively, we've all known a great deal about the nature of emotions for a long time. After meeting someone new we've all heard people say, "The chemistry is right," or "There just wasn't any chemistry between us." They could be talking about meeting the great love of their life, or applying for a job. Intuitively, we recognize that apparently intangible and invisible factors stir in our bodies.

The emotional link to the physical is clear. When we're frightened our emotional reaction may be to break out in a cold sweat, our knees may wobble and our mouths go dry, chills may run up and down our spines, or we may break out in goose bumps.

When we're angry our faces may flush; when we're nervous we may sweat a lot and our hands may feel clammy. The chemistry within our bodies comes to a boil; we may think these powerful feelings will overwhelm us unless we keep them under wraps. No wonder we often try to hide or ignore our emotions.

But to be emotionally tough—a key element in every kind of success—we need to learn how to control our emotions through a toughening adaptation. Emotions are based on body chemistry, not on "that old black magic." Understanding this fact is the first step toward emotional toughening.

Biochemical Adaptation

Some of the most exciting and insightful research into this area deals with the biochemistry of stress and specifically with the biochemistry of emotion. Later we will explore in greater detail the basic understanding that emotions are biochemical events. Fear, joy, anger, and responses to threat or challenge are all emotions that have different neurochemical and neuroendocrine foundations. The fact that drugs such as cocaine, morphine, heroin, alcohol, and tranquilizers can powerfully affect mood and emotion supports the view that emotional reactions have a biochemical basis.

Physiological Toughness

The physiological toughness model developed by Richard Dienstbier of the University of Nebraska also supports this view. Dienstbier strongly contends that physical and emotional toughening has a clear biochemical basis. His toughening model, which

will also be given a more detailed review later, asserts that toughness is the result of neuroendocrine changes stemming from intermittent actions during cycles of stress. According to Dienstbier,
these neuroendocrine changes are linked to both positive performance and emotional stability.

Neurochemical Adaptations

As early as 1975, researchers began exploring the connection between emotion and various neurochemicals such as endorphins,
neuropeptides, and neurotransmitters. Candace Pert, former chief
of brain biochemistry at the National Institute of Mental Health,
has devoted much of her career to studying how brain chemicals
such as endorphins control emotion. Years of investigation have
convinced Pert that neuropeptides—small, proteinlike chemicals
concentrated in the brain's limbic system—are the biochemical
manifestation of emotion.

, The limbic system has long been known to be the brain's emotional center, controlling everything from the catecholamines, the
chemicals involved in the stress response, to the neurohormones
that affect heart rate, sex drive, and other emotional responses.
Pert believes that one day neuroscience will link specific emotional
states to specific blood chemicals. We may discover that each of the
states of feeling that we know as an emotion—anger, fear, pleasure,
and so on—has a unique chemical profile, much as the training
process of a muscle has a specific chemical profile.

Indirect support for Pert's neurochemical work also comes
from a new area of research—psychoneuroimmunology (PNI),
which explores the effect of brain function and brain chemistry on
immune cells. PNI research has shown that the brain and the immune system are directly linked, and that communication works
both ways between them.

Increasing amounts of evidence support the conclusion that
the chemical components of thought and emotion can actually ener-
gize the immune system or shut it down. PNI research is helping
us understand how and why overstressed people get sick, and why
emotionally strong, positive people often have more effective immune systems. In Chapter 11 we will learn how to toughen our immune systems by applying the same principles of toughening used
to strengthen us physically and emotionally.

Physical and emotional stress share common biochemical and neurochemical foundations, and because of this, physical toughening often leads to automatic increases in emotional toughening. Similarly, emotional toughening generally brings about a higher level of physical toughness.

Everything we do has energy expenditure and energy recovery properties. Life itself can be viewed in terms of expending and recapturing energy. For those reasons, balancing stress and recovery on a daily basis is essential for achieving maximum happiness and health.

To live is to oscillate; to die is to cease to oscillate. Living things pulsate; nonliving things (except mechanical gadgets) do not. Even at the cellular level, the pulsating rhythms of stress and recovery are evident. Breathing, heart rate (EKG), brain waves (EEG), and muscle activity (EMG) are observable wave forms of energy expenditure and recovery. Highly linear episodes of stress are dysfunctional, as are highly linear episodes of recovery. Unfortunately, life today is so stressful that it works powerfully against opportunities for energy recovery.

THE HEALTHY ART OF MAKING WAVES

One final reason for accepting that emotional toughening is a neurochemical and biochemical adaptation is the work of Irv Dardik, who served for seven years as the founding chairman of the United States Olympic Committee's Sports Medicine Council. Dardik based his work on Nobel Prize winner Llya Priogogine's discovery that molecules communicate when they are oscillating. After years of studying the human heart under stress, Dardik has developed a wave-energy theory of disease that has far-reaching scientific implications.

Dardik contends that rhythmic waves of stress and recovery promote disease reversal. Prolonged linear episodes of either excessive stress or excessive recovery decrease the ability of our immune systems to ward off disease. According to Dardik, balanced cycles of stress and rest activate the body's repair processes and immune chemistry in positive ways and strengthen the person's emotional and physical capacity to manage future stress. In other words, balanced cycles of stress and recovery stabilize the body's delicate biochemical and neurochemical interactions.

Dardik states that producing intermittent cycles of physical stress followed by cycles of balanced recovery—what he refers to as "making waves"—is the critical element in rebuilding and strengthening the immune system. With his patients, Dardik produces waves of stress and recovery through physical exercise; he uses rising and falling heart rates as indicators of balanced and unbalanced cycles.

Making waves is another term for the same concept of balance between the stress and recovery cycles we've been discussing. Whether we express it as day and night, peaks and valleys, or ebb and flow, the recurring themes of toughening always involve dynamic movement, expansion of challenge, change, growth, oscillation, and rhythm alternating with rest and recovery.

Although Dardik's work and theory focused primarily on the disease process and specifically on the reversal of chronic disease, his wave-energy theory supported what I had discovered in my work in toughening athletes. His theory and work with diseased patients strongly reinforced my findings regarding the role of stress and recovery in health and performance. Where Dardik had seen the value of making waves as a means of reversing disease, I had independently discovered the powerful role balanced stress and recovery play in the toughening process.

WHEN YOU FORCE YOUR BODY
TO MAKE THE WAVES

If you don't create waves naturally, your body will find a way to get your chemistry moving—possibly by the use of killer drugs such as nicotine, cocaine, or crack, or the abusive overuse of caffeine, alcohol, or food. Eating disorders such as anorexia and bulimia are misguided attempts to create powerful waves of stress and recovery.

Severe depressive disorders such as catatonia—characterized by total withdrawal, muscular rigidity, and stupor—represent conditions of extreme linearity. In such cases, the stress/recovery relationship freezes in time because the victim's biochemistry has stopped oscillating. Even today, electroconvulsive therapy is one of the few successful intervention strategies for catatonia. A massive jolt of stress electricity shocks the patient's biochemistry into making a powerful wave of its own.

Manic depressive disorders represent another misguided answer to the body's desperate search for a way to keep its biochemistry moving. In these cases, individuals oscillate between periods of manic activity and arousal, and extreme depression and withdrawal. Each complete manic depressive cycle represents a stress/recovery wave, albeit one that is antisocial, dangerous, or even criminal.

The point is brutally simple and clear. If we don't find healthy, natural ways to oscillate—to live balanced lives—the response our body forces on us is very likely to be destructive or even tragic.

HOW IS A BALANCED LIFE ACHIEVED?

Traditional wisdom teaches that a balanced life is a healthy life, but how that occurs and what that means have remained largely philosophical matters. Moving from philosophy to practicality, the Toughness Training for Life system will illustrate how issues such as drive, motivation, achievement, self-esteem, and even personal happiness itself are directly linked to the harmonious interaction of balanced stress and recovery cycles.

SUMMARY

- **Toughening occurs** in response to periodic exposure to progressively increasing cycles of physical and/or emotional stress alternating with regular periods of recovery. This process is called Toughness Training.
- **Weakening occurs** in response to:
  - Repeated exposure to cycles of excessive stress and insufficient recovery, known as overtraining.
  - Repeated exposure to cycles of insufficient stress and excessive recovery, known as undertraining.

- **Maximum health, happiness, and productivity occur** when:
  - Sufficient physical and emotional toughness are acquired to effectively manage the volume of stress in one's life.
  - Balanced cycles of stress and recovery are consistently created in as many areas of life as possible. A healthy, happy, productive life is filled with stimulation, punctuated by balanced recovery.

3

BOTH OVERTRAINING

AND UNDERTRAINING

CAN DAMAGE YOUR LIFE

FATIGUE

BOREDOM

INSOMNIA

LAZINESS

ANNOYANCE

MOODINESS

LOW ENERGY

IRRITATION

LOW MOTIVATION

WEIGHT PROBLEMS

POOR CONCENTRATION

DECLINING PRODUCTIVITY

REDUCED SENSE OF HUMOR

PHYSICAL ACHES AND PAINS

EATING/APPETITE PROBLEMS

DIMINISHED WORK ENJOYMENT

FREQUENT COLD AND FLU SYMPTOMS

INCREASINGLY NEGATIVE ATTITUDE

AMPLIFIED ANXIETY AND NERVOUSNESS

POOR AND INCONSISTENT PERFORMANCE

MAGNIFIED SENSE OF PRESSURE AND STRESS

Do these symptoms sound familiar? As varied as they may seem, they all have significant links to excessive work and also to excessive rest in life, as well as being linked to over- and undertraining in sport.

HOW MUCH IS TOO MUCH?

Determining how much stress athletes can take is one of the greatest challenges in coaching. If pushed too hard, athletes deteriorate; if not pushed enough, they never reach their full potential. Coaching decisions concerning when, how much, and how long to push literally make or break an athlete's chances for success. When coaches err, it's almost always in the direction of overtraining, because today's sport world is so dominated by the win-at-any-cost, no-pain-no-gain philosophy.

Many performance problems have been presented to me in the past 16 years as burnout, lack of confidence, poor concentration, broken spirit, choking response, and low motivation. However, more than 75 percent of them were related importantly to emotional overtraining, physical overtraining, or both.

Decisions about when, how much, and how long to push also make or break people in business careers outside of sport. The consequences of overtraining and undertraining in ordinary life are just as real and evident as they are in the highly visible world of professional sport. Wherever encountered, excessive or insufficient stress can severely limit—or even enormously diminish—happiness, health, and productivity.

However, a critical difference exists here between the sport and nonsport worlds. In sport the greatest risk is physical overtraining and emotional overtraining; in nonsport life, it's physical *under*training and emotional overtraining. Before going further, let's review precisely what overtraining and undertraining are in sport and life.

Overtraining occurs when the volume of stress—physical or emotional—exceeds the limit the individual can handle. That limit is referred to as one's adaptation threshold. In ordinary life, overlimit stress is excessive work.

Undertraining occurs when the volume of stress is insufficient for the desired adaptation to take place—in daily life, too much rest. This is commonly seen in the loss of fitness experienced by sedentary people, and similarly, in the stunted personalities and declining mental capabilities of people who avoid all kinds of new interests and intellectual challenges.

Overtraining is too much stress; undertraining is too little stress. Both problems are conditions of imbalance. Figure 3.1 is a graphic representation of balanced stress and recovery.

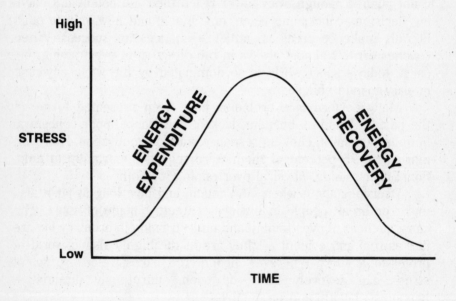

Figure 3.1   Stress and Recovery in Balance

Here the energy expended is fully recaptured during the recovery period. When stress and recovery are balanced, the risk of overtraining can be ignored. But when stress levels exceed an individual's adaptation limits, recovery mechanisms fail, and overtraining's serious consequences follow.

Similarly, when energy recovery exceeds energy expenditure for an extended period, the erosions of undertraining take place.

Physically this means a decline in fitness, and may involve weight gain and muscle loss as well. If the undertraining extends into the mental and emotional areas of life, losses in mental acuity and emotional toughness take place. As seen in Figure 3.2, overtraining and undertraining represent opposing ends of the same stress continuum.

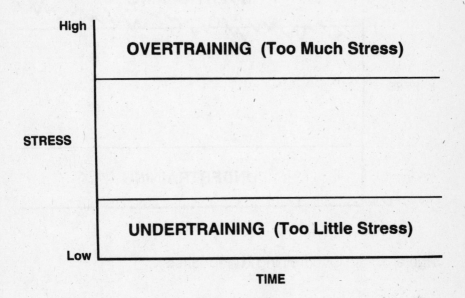

Figure 3.2   The Continuum of Stress

In the Toughness Training model, overtraining, overstress, excessive stress, excessive energy expenditure, and overwork all mean the same thing: nonadaptive episodes of too much stress. Similarly, undertraining, understress, insufficient stress, insufficient energy expenditure, lack of challenge, and excessive rest refer to nonadaptive episodes of too little stress.

Figure 3.3 illustrates classic overtraining. Here the volume of stress is extremely high and linear for a long time—that is, in a nearly straight line with only minor variations. Linear stress occurs when energy expenditure is not balanced by recovery.

In Figure 3.4, an illustration of classic undertraining, the volume of stress is low and linear. When energy recovery is not balanced by stress, no gain in capacity will occur, a condition known as linear recovery.

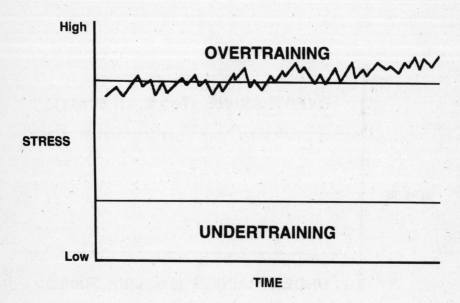

Figure 3.3   Overtraining (Linear Stress)

Both overtraining and undertraining can be viewed as not enough or too much recovery. The old saying "All work and no play makes Jack a dull boy" is balanced by a newer truism, "All play and no work makes Jack useless."

Avoiding mental effort for long periods will prevent Jack from functioning at his intellectual peak. His emotional toughness is likely to decline as well. On top of all this, if Jack doesn't get much exercise during his rest binges, his physical condition will also deteriorate.

The greatest risk of overtraining occurs when high stress continues for extended periods without interludes of recovery. An example of this in the emotional arena is someone experiencing constant fear because of financial pressure for many weeks without relief.

Surprisingly, overtraining can occur when stress levels are not high—if they continue for a long time unrelieved by recovery. This is to say that normal, moderate stress can eventually become excessive if recovery is inadequate over time. This happens when energy reserves are exhausted because the supply of available energy has slowly declined below what is adequate for moderate stress.

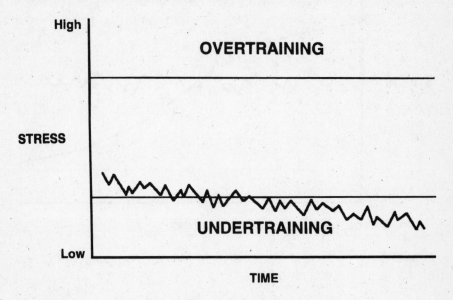

Figure 3.4   Undertraining (Linear Recovery)

An important understanding here is that the closer an individual comes to exhausting his or her energy reserves, the less tolerance that person has for energy expenditure—for additional effort of any kind. The risk of overtraining increases as normal stress gradually approaches excessive stress.

A good example of this in the physical arena is what happens to overworked muscles. A man who runs ten miles although trained for only two will likely find his leg muscles start to fail (cramping, muscle tears, failure to contract properly, and so on). What was moderate or even low stress for two miles becomes excessive stress before ten miles are run. As glycogen and energy stores in the leg muscles are depleted, the muscles begin to lose their tolerance for energy expenditure. Figure 3.5 illustrates this scenario:

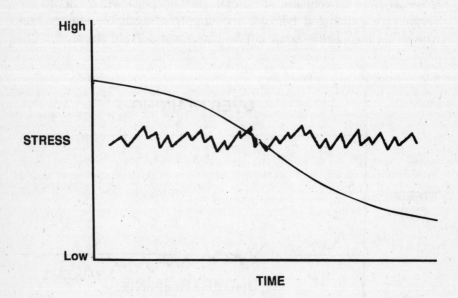

Figure 3.5   Without Recovery, All Stress Eventually Becomes Excessive Stress

STRESS AND TOUGHNESS TRAINING

One of the most important understandings this book offers is that both overtraining and undertraining weaken rather than toughen. With overtraining, the intensity, duration, or overall volume of stress is so great that it destroys rather than builds. With undertraining, the intensity, duration, or overall volume of stress is too low to cause adaptation (toughening).

Overtraining weakens by damaging and reducing flexibility, responsiveness, strength, and resiliency. Undertraining weakens in two ways: first, by failing to maintain current levels of toughness; second, by failing to offset time's slow deterioration.

Clearly, the volume of stress that toughens must lie somewhere between the extremes of overtraining and undertraining. As we learned in Chapter 2, we get tougher by progressively challenging ourselves beyond our normal limits. However, many of us, either deliberately or unconsciously, adopt a maintenance stress program. This means we keep ourselves on a steady course as to stress and recovery and merely maintain our current toughness level.

HOW TOUGHENING HAPPENS

There are four types of stress, and only one leads to toughening. Excessive stress and insufficient stress actually decrease toughness, while maintenance stress freezes it at current levels. As shown in Figure 3.6, only adaptive stress toughens.

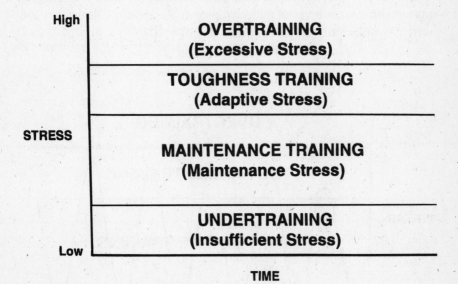

Figure 3.6   The Only One That Toughens

You have several choices in getting tougher. You can embark on Toughness Training simultaneously in all three spheres—physical, emotional, and mental—or you can take one on at a time.

In choosing your Toughness Training program, consider (1) your current level of emotional toughness, (2) the sphere in which you need greater toughness soonest, and (3) the energy you can devote to increasing your toughness and capability to win life's battles more often.

Whatever your decision, you will need to learn how to recognize and control the various levels of personal stress. Equally important, you'll need to learn how to provide yourself with adequate recovery. In making your plans, bear in mind that you will also need to follow a consistent program that progressively increases stress in the sphere or spheres you choose for toughening. A great deal of guidance on these matters is given in later chapters.

Figure 3.7 shows that toughening results from exposure to periods of stress that progressively extend you beyond your normal limits and then allow you to fully recapture the lost energy. The ideal process of toughening gradually builds over time after beginning at the lowest level of adaptive stress (to avoid pushing you too hard too fast—and probably into discouragement or injury).

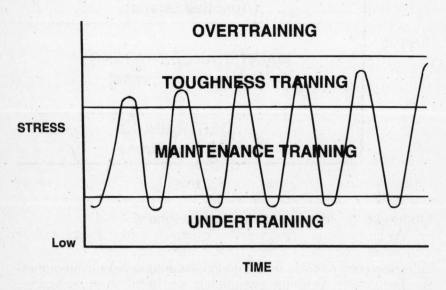

Figure 3.7   Cycles That Toughen

As you get tougher, your capacity for managing cycles of stress will broaden. As seen in Figure 3.8, your range of coping steadily increases as you get tougher. This simply means that you can effectively manage more stress. Just the opposite occurs with weakening, as shown in Figure 3.9.

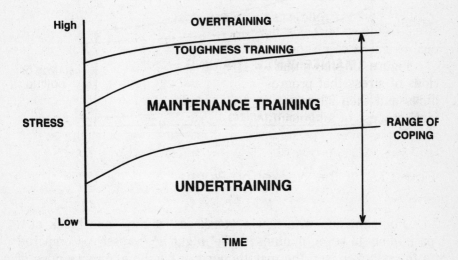

Figure 3.8   The Toughening Process

It's important to understand that as you toughen, your range of coping increases. The more stress you can handle, the more stress you need to maintain or you'll start to lose it. This applies to all three spheres: physical, mental, and emotional stress.

As an example, let's compare a marathon runner to someone who never exercises. If well trained, the marathoner can run 26 miles at a pace of six to seven minutes a mile without incurring excessive stress. The volume of training needed to maintain this capacity is maintenance training. Anything greater would be either

Toughness Training or overtraining; anything less would be undertraining.

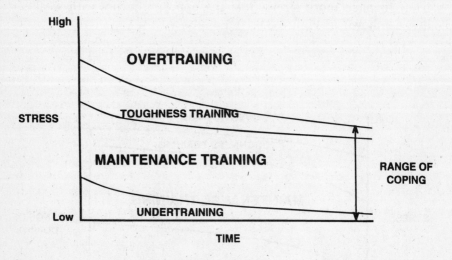

Figure 3.9   The Weakening Process

For someone who never exercises, running one block at a pace of six to seven minutes a mile might be excessive. Compared to the nonexerciser, the marathoner can handle a massive dose of physical stress. However, a consistently high volume of stress (distance running in this case) is required to maintain that level of toughness—to avoid undertraining. The nonexerciser must begin training at a very low level of physical stress to avoid overtraining and its consequent weakening. What would be overtraining for the marathoner might be serious—even dangerous—overtraining for the nonexerciser.

As Figures 3.8 and 3.9 also show, at the extremes the band of stress separating maintenance training from overtraining decreases. At the extremes—marathon training on the high end and no training on the low end—it becomes increasingly difficult to distinguish between stress that toughens (adaptive) and stress that weakens (overtraining or undertraining). At either extreme, even a slight increase in stress might be too much.

The same is true emotionally. An individual who is able to effectively manage a high volume of stress must continue to experience this volume to avoid emotional weakening. The range of coping for someone who is emotionally strong is very broad. For someone who is emotionally weak, it is very narrow.

LISTENING TO THE LANGUAGE OF PAIN

Distinguishing between insufficient stress and maintenance stress—and also between adaptive stress and excessive stress—is a vital toughening skill. Learn how. It's primarily a matter of grasping what the four kinds of stress are, and paying keen attention to determine what kind you're under as you participate in your various activities.

Low stress usually is enjoyable for short periods of time; it allows the temporary recovery of energy associated with feelings of relief. However, when low stress becomes chronic or excessive, emotional pain in the form of boredom, low motivation, laziness, depression, confusion, or apathy often emerges.

Since maintenance stress is your normal stress load, you are likely to feel stimulated but not uncomfortable. Remember, however, that a very comfortable volume of physical or emotional stress for you may be serious overtraining that's much too powerful for someone else.

KEY POINT:

YOUR IDEAL PERFORMANCE STATE WILL

LIKELY OCCUR TOWARD THE UPPER RANGE

OF MAINTENANCE STRESS.

You'll feel stimulated, comfortable, and positive. You'll still be performing within yourself, not feeling overly pushed or excessively challenged. Feelings of pressure will be minimal.

Adaptive stress pushes you beyond your normal limits. The volume of stress is highly challenging, and is accompanied by feelings of discomfort. You feel pushed, pressured, vulnerable. You can feel you're beyond your comfort zone, but the level of discomfort is manageable. If you're not feeling pushed or pressured, the volume of stress is not likely to lead to toughening.

Real pain is the consequence of excessive stress. Elite athletes become very skillful at distinguishing between the normal discomfort associated with progressive training and real pain. Pain is a signal to stop! As we'll see, the pain associated with excessive stress can be physical, emotional, or mental.

As the volume of stress is turned up and down, the body is always sending signals of how it is coping with the energy expenditure. To avoid both undertraining and overtraining and to consistently expose ourselves to levels of stress that will toughen us, we must learn to read the body's stress signals. We must listen to the language of pain and understand the message.

Let's briefly review what we know about overtraining and undertraining:

- Overtraining and undertraining in sport are analogous to excessive work and excessive rest in life.
- Overtraining and undertraining represent opposing ends of the same stress continuum.
- Overtraining is too much work/stress and too little recovery over time.
- Undertraining is too little work/stress and too much recovery over time.
- Stress that toughens (adaptive stress) falls between maintenance stress and excessive stress.
- Overtraining and undertraining decrease your range of coping, which is the volume of stress you can manage effectively.
- Stress is physical, mental, and emotional.

HARDER THAN IT LOOKS

The total volume of stress an individual experiences is the sum of physical, mental, and emotional energy that he or she burns at any given moment. For this reason, distinguishing between physical stress, mental stress, and emotional stress is critical to our understanding of undertraining and overtraining.

At first glance, it looks easy. Defining physical stress as the physical body's energy expenditure and mental and emotional stress as the nonphysical body's energy expenditure might initially seem quite plausible. The difficulty is that thoughts and feelings are measurable, tangible neurochemical events as real as the physical body's actions. Just as physical stress produces physical changes in muscles (EMG), brain activity (EEG), and heart rate (EKG), so too does mental and emotional stress.

When you sprint 20 yards, muscle tension and heartbeat increase dramatically. Fear and anger produce nearly identical physical reactions. The plain fact is that distinguishing physical, mental, and emotional stress on a physical/nonphysical basis simply doesn't work.

OUTSIDE-IN STRESS

For purposes of this model, physical stress is energy expended by the musculoskeletal system in the form of work or play. Working out is physical; it involves muscle movement that leads to a variety of internal changes. Therefore, physical stress—running, jumping, walking, sitting, and so on—is outside-in.

INSIDE-OUT STRESS

Thoughts and feelings begin inside the skull as neurochemical events that can lead to any number of outer changes in the physical body. In other words, they move from the brain outward. Thinking, feeling, concentrating, perceiving, and so on are inside-out forms of energy expenditure.

It's also useful to differentiate mental from emotional stress. Mental stress is energy expended in the nonemotional processing of sensed information and ideas in perceiving, thinking, concentrating, and so forth. Emotional stress is energy expended in the expression of one's feelings. Thinking about how to get to your dentist's office is mental stress; fearing what happens when you get there is emotional stress.

Emotional stress levels are generally much higher than mental stress levels; negative emotional states usually burn more energy than positive emotional states do. Typically, you'll spend more energy worrying about a dental appointment than feeling excited about going to the movies.

Because both mental and emotional stress are inside-out stress forms, and because most emotional stress is closely tied to positive and negative thinking patterns, references to emotional stress in this book generally include mental stress as well. When it's important to distinguish between emotional and nonemotional stress, the term "mental stress" will be used.

―――――――― **SYMPTOMS OF OVERTRAINING AND UNDERTRAINING** ――――――――

The body has its own unique ways of signaling when it's overworked or underworked. Grasping this reality marked a great breakthrough for me that significantly changed my interpretation of what I was hearing both inside and outside of sport.

I realized that what had been called problems of laziness and poor attitude were clearly something else. I came to understand that expressions of fatigue, negative emotions, low motivation, or moodiness did not reflect character flaws or personality weaknesses any more than physical pain does.

People aren't poorly motivated or bored because they are lazy. Problems of fatigue, poor concentration, or low enjoyment aren't resolved by simply trying harder. It's natural and a sign of good health to be motivated, passionate, and positively energized. To lack these qualities means that something is wrong either physically, emotionally, or in both spheres.

―――――――― **COPING WITH LOW ENERGY AND LOW MOTIVATION** ――――――――

It became clear that reduced motivation was often the body's way of protecting itself from the ravages of overtraining. If you're unmotivated, you're not as likely to overdo it physically or emotionally. Only when stress and recovery are in balance does the mind and body realize that it can safely work harder. When this happens, passion returns.

Attributing problems of low motivation and low energy to laziness and poor effort is counterproductive. That approach does nothing positive; on the negative side it perpetuates and intensifies highly destructive feelings of guilt, confusion, and self-doubt.

Surprisingly, the symptoms of overtraining and undertraining are quite similar. Both include mental, physical, and emotional signs.

OVERTRAINING AND UNDERTRAINING SYMPTOMS

MENTAL	EMOTIONAL	PHYSICAL
Fatigue	Fatigue	Fatigue
Laziness	Laziness	Laziness
Low energy	Low energy	Low energy
Poor performance	Poor performance	Poor performance
Poor concentration	Irritation	Eating problems
Negative thinking	Less enjoyment	Muscle tightness
Confusion	and fun	Sleep problems
Poor problem-solving	Boredom	Suppressed immune
	Low motivation	system
	Moodiness	Overweight prob-
	Anxiety	lems
	Reduced humor	Underweight prob-
		lems

SYMPTOM SUMMARY

Here are a few things I've come to understand about symptoms in relation to Toughness Training:

- Fatigue, boredom, low energy, and poor motivation often signal that stress is excessive. More directly, they protect to some degree against further overtraining, energy expenditure, and stress, whether the stress being defended against is mental, emotional, or physical.
- Fatigue, boredom, low energy, and poor motivation can also signal too little stimulation (stress) and too much recovery.
- Concentration problems and negative thinking almost always accompany stress/recovery problems.
- Increased irritability, moodiness, and negative emotion are common signs of overtraining.

- Increased anxiety, nervousness, and worry often reflect stress/recovery problems.
- Energy recovery mechanisms often fail under conditions of excessive stress. (This is one of the most important findings of all. A good example is sleep. During periods of excessive stress, it seems reasonable that people will sleep better because they need it more. Unfortunately, the opposite usually happens. Sleep problems often indicate overtraining.)
- Unbalanced stress/recovery cycles disrupt the body's biological clocks, as various appetite problems show. Hunger at inopportune times and craving the wrong foods are common symptoms of both undertraining and overtraining.
- Body weight problems such as binging and purging food often indicate overtraining, particularly for women.
- The mental, emotional, and physical signs of overtraining and undertraining are very similar.
- Excessive physical stress can lead to mental or emotional problems. This is very common among athletes, where physical stress proceeds from the muscles inward, eventually interacting with the same systems that affect thoughts and emotions (nervous system, neuroendocrine system, and so on).
- Excessive emotional stress can lead to physical or mental problems. Emotional stress triggers a chain of biochemical events within the brain that instantly influence thinking and proceed outward from the brain to the body. Cardiovascular, neuromuscular, and immune systems are affected. This is a very common scenario in everyday life.
- Excessive mental stress can lead to physical and emotional problems. However, because purely mental stress burns far less energy than physical or emotional stress, it causes the fewest overtraining problems. Few people are overtraining (overstressed) in all three spheres—mental, emotional, and physical—at the same time. More commonly an individual is overstressed in one sphere and understressed in another, and suffers the consequences of both extremes simultaneously. The next section deals with these matters.

CASE HISTORIES OF
OVERTRAINING/UNDERTRAINING SYNDROMES

We will now look at concrete examples of overtraining and undertraining. An actual case study of a real person (names changed) is provided for each of four categories.

—— 1. UNDERTRAINING PHYSICALLY, OVERTRAINING EMOTIONALLY ——

John, age 42; division head of a large petroleum company; married with two children, ages 9 and 11.

Presenting Complaints

Weight gain (15 pounds in three months and already 50 pounds overweight); wakes up tired and feels constant fatigue throughout the day; unable to fall asleep at night although exhausted. John's motivation has declined; he is more irritable, feels constant pressure, and says he can never relax or wind down. His job satisfaction and enjoyment are decreasing.

John has recurring cold and flu symptoms, and fears he may have a serious health problem although a recent comprehensive medical exam revealed only two concerns: slightly high blood pressure and the excessive weight. John feels disconnected from his family and guilty that he doesn't spend more time with them.

Typical Day

Up at 6:45 A.M. No breakfast; a minimum of three cups of coffee before leaving home. The normal drive to work takes one hour and 15 minutes, longer with heavy traffic. Usually has a high-fat snack with a diet soda between 10:30 and 11:00. At 1:00, John takes a 30-minute lunch break; afterward he works until 6:00 P.M.

Workdays are stressful and intense. He generally arrives home by 7:30 P.M., watches TV until dinner at 8:00 P.M., which is usually a large, high-fat meal. John then spends 30 to 45 minutes reviewing office materials and finishes the day watching TV. Often falls asleep on the couch and awakens to the TV blaring. Usually in bed by midnight.

John's only exercise is occasional weekend golf, and after-dinner walks with his wife about twice a month. He spends Sunday trying to catch up on work, resting, and sleeping.

Comments

In these times, both men and women are at high risk for undertraining physically and overtraining emotionally. Most so afflicted fall into a pattern of decreasing motion and increasing emotion.

A continuous barrage of emotional stressors pounds people today. Persistent, consuming, and often conflicting career, family, and financial pressures can cause highly linear cycles of emotional stress.

The reverse is often true physically. Office workers remain virtually motionless all day—sitting, standing, waiting. Without periodic spikes of movement and exercise, their bodies are chronically understimulated. And because of their high emotional stress, many feel too exhausted to exercise after work. Quite simply, they don't feel like moving.

When exercise is not used to break these high cycles of emotional stress, many people rely on food or on alcohol or other drugs for relief from linearity. This generates some emotional recovery, but at enormous physical cost, because overindulgence in food or drugs often becomes habitual, addictive, and harmful in itself. In any case such addictions increase linearity, frequently to an extremely dangerous degree.

John's physical undertraining and emotional overtraining have made him weaker in both areas. His symptoms are classic, resulting in less flexibility, responsiveness, strength, and resiliency under stress. Most important for John, his sharply lowered toughness clearly has reduced his happiness, health, and productivity.

—— **2. OVERTRAINING PHYSICALLY, UNDERTRAINING EMOTIONALLY** ——

Jim, age 33; dockworker; married; one child, age 5.

Presenting Complaints

Constant physical aches and pains; chronic soreness in right shoulder (rotator cuff tendinitis); persistent fatigue; low motivation; boredom; low work enjoyment; low productivity; sleep irregularities.

Moody and quick to anger, Jim drinks a minimum of six beers after work, and occasionally binges.

Typical Day

Up at 7:30 A.M. Large breakfast. Drives thirty minutes to his job. Works 9:00 to 6:00 with one hour for lunch. (Jim takes his lunch and sleeps at least 30 minutes during the lunch hour.) His job involves loading and unloading ship cargo not accessible to heavy equipment. The work is physically demanding but nonstimulating emotionally. According to Jim, the days seem to drag on forever, particularly the late-afternoon hours, when boredom, fatigue, and nagging shoulder pain set in.

Jim arrives home exhausted and emotionally distant. He immediately opens his first beer and collapses on the TV couch. At 7:30 he eats a large dinner that's usually high in fat, after which he returns to the TV and continues drinking.

Jim's wife understands his need for rest and distance and, although she does her best to help, feels extreme loneliness and anger at Jim's lack of affection and attention. She reports several bitter arguments in the past month.

Comments

This syndrome usually strikes people with physically demanding but boring jobs. The at-risk group for it includes certain types of factory workers, farm workers, assembly-line workers, manual laborers, and pieceworkers.

Even people in such outwardly glamorous jobs as teaching tennis or aerobic dance can incur this syndrome because of the repetitious nature of their work and its extreme physical demands.

Jim's personal happiness, health, and productivity are being seriously undermined by this tragic—and, sadly, quite frequent—combination of high linear physical stress and low linear emotional stress. Jim continues to weaken, becoming increasingly less flexible, responsive, strong, and resilient, both physically and emotionally. Jim's use of alcohol has become his primary way to break the linear cycles of emotional and physical stress that are crushing his life.

—— **3.** UNDERTRAINING PHYSICALLY, UNDERTRAINING EMOTIONALLY ——

Mary, age 53; married with one child, age 23, no longer living at home. Formerly a dental assistant, Mary hasn't worked for five years.

Presenting Complaints

Low self-esteem; low energy; constantly tired; has difficulty waking up in the morning (reports she could sleep all day). Mary gained 26 pounds in the last six months, is now 65 pounds overweight. A compulsive overeater with an extremely low tolerance for stress of any kind, Mary cries easily and often. Her husband is deeply concerned about her periods of depression, moodiness, and unhappiness.

Typical Day

Up between 10:00 and noon. Coffee and juice for breakfast (drinks as many as ten cups of caffeinated coffee per day). Spends most of the afternoon watching TV sitcoms and soap operas, reading magazines, and cooking. Mary doesn't exercise; in fact, she never leaves home if she can avoid it. Although she eats very little during the day, she usually has three or four cocktails in the evening with her husband before they begin their large dinner at 8:00 P.M. Mary watches movies until 1:00 or 2:00 A.M., often snacking on sweets after her husband falls asleep. She occasionally leaves home to buy groceries, but feels uncomfortable doing so (reports that going outside the home without her husband is becoming increasingly stressful).

Comments

Mary is a classic example of someone overly protected from physical and emotional stress. Because of her avoidance of all stress—interacting with people, fighting traffic, moving, exercising, and so forth—her ability to manage any stress at all is rapidly vanishing. Along with a severely reduced range of coping with stress, her self-esteem and self-confidence have also declined seriously.

In the physical sphere, Mary's chronic state of linear recovery is progressively destroying her capacity to expend energy—that is, to do anything at all. She has limited her emotional stimulation to

TV sitcoms and soap operas, and to food and alcohol—to an extent that may have reached the addictive level. Although Mary's consumption of food and alcohol give her temporary relief from her escalating feelings of inadequacy, it compounds her chronic problems with recovery.

In her own misguided way, Mary is trying to create balanced cycles of stress and recovery. Her progression, which follows a fairly common path, goes as follows.

Boredom and depression (low energy) are temporarily broken by emotional excitement from TV soap operas. Although that source increases her abnormally low energy level slightly and delivers some temporary relief from her extreme linearity, the lack of real emotional stimulation allows Mary's depression and fear to quickly return.

In the evening, alcohol gives Mary some temporary relief from her negative stressors. However, since alcohol depresses the central nervous system and decreases energy and arousal, it provides only a short-lived and unsatisfactory form of recovery. Mary then moves to compulsive eating for its waves of pleasure and relief from linearity that are quickly smothered by larger waves of depression, fear, and guilt.

—— **4. OVERTRAINING PHYSICALLY, OVERTRAINING EMOTIONALLY** ——

Todd, age 15; junior tennis player with high Florida ranking.

Presenting Complaints

Poor performance in last few tournaments; low motivation, poor concentration; constantly fatigued; low energy on court; weight loss (seven pounds in two months); accused of being "lazy" by coach and parents; reduced enjoyment of tennis and school; more negative and self-critical; diminished fighting spirit on court.

Todd constantly complains about muscle soreness, muscle pulls, and other physical aches and pains (his coach and parents interpret these excuses as simply part of his laziness); his school grades, formerly all A's, now include B's and C's.

Typical Day

Up at 6:15. Eats breakfast about twice a week. (His mother encourages Todd to have breakfast every day, but he's usually not hungry and doesn't want to eat.) In school from 7:15 to 12:30, a special mornings-only schedule for children attending tennis academy. At lunch, 12:45 to 1:15, Todd usually eats very little; he doesn't like the academy food, which is often very high in fat and protein. Tennis, 1:30 to 4:30; physical conditioning, 4:30 to 5:30; private coaching on strokes and tactics, 5:30 to 6:15; dinner, 7:00; homework, 7:30 to 9:30. Three out of five weekends Todd plays tournaments.

Todd complains that he has no time for himself and that he feels constant pressure from his parents to excel in both school and tennis. Todd's mother attends all his tennis practice sessions, takes notes, and coaches him from the sides of the court. Both parents frequently voice their opinion that Todd is being lazy and undisciplined, and are frustrated and angry with him because he refuses to work hard enough to turn things around. As a result, they have taken away some of his privileges with his friends (parties, movies, and so forth) until he improves his grades and attitude on the tennis court.

Comments

Todd is now 17 and no longer plays tennis. He hasn't had any desire to step onto a court in over seven months. His perplexed, angry parents continue to believe that Todd's withdrawal from tennis is simple laziness and poor self-discipline. In reality, Todd's withdrawal was the only way his mind and body could break the destructive cycle of emotional and physical linearity. Although not a conscious decision, his burnout and motivational collapse were the only way he could obtain the relief and sustained recovery he desperately needed. As we'll discover in later chapters, motivation is a great barometer of the vital balance between stress and recovery.

Too much stress or too little stress decreases motivation. "Laziness" more often than not is a stress/recovery problem, not a character weakness or a personality defect.

Clearly, the extreme emotional and physical linearity of Todd's competitive tennis training has weakened him. The signs of overtraining were everywhere in Todd's life; however, his parents, teachers, and coach didn't see or understand them, or they misinterpreted them altogether. The consequences for Todd have been severe: reduced happiness, health, and productivity. He continues to be less flexible, responsive, strong, and resilient under stress.

FUN IS THE BEST ANSWER

The best single measure of the balance of stress and recovery in your life is pure positive energy: fun. As the amount of negative stress in your life increases, your sense of fun and joy tends to decrease—although you don't have to let this happen. (In later chapters we'll discuss how you can avoid this dangerous loss of fun and joy in positive, nondestructive ways.)

Fun means excitement and arousal (energy expenditure) without physical or psychological pain (negative stress). The more you love an activity and continue to have fun doing it, the lower your risk of overtraining.

KEY POINT:

WHEN THE FUN STOPS, PAY ATTENTION;

PAIN IS PROBABLY NOT FAR BEHIND.

4

RECOVERY TRAINING—

YOUR MISSING LINK?

KAROSHI

It's a Japanese word.

Death *(shi)* from overwork *(karo)*.

Karoshi is becoming more common in Japan as men and women struggle to meet the physical and emotional demands of modern Japanese life. Long work hours, little or no exercise, constant pressure to meet expectations, relentless traffic, little time for family, too much alcohol, too many cigarettes, increasing financial pressures, and a poor diet set the stage. The curtain comes down, not from an acute episode of *karo* (overwork), not from an epidemic of some insidious *karo* virus, but from heart attacks, complications of high blood pressure, lung cancer, suicide, and the entire collection of degenerative diseases.

Research conducted by Japan's Institute of Public Health identified five patterns of work that lead to the fatal *karoshi* syndrome:

1. Extremely long hours that interfere with normal recovery and rest patterns
2. Night work that interferes with normal recovery and rest patterns
3. Working without holidays or breaks
4. High-pressure work without breaks
5. Extremely demanding physical labor and continuously stressful work without relief

Significantly, inadequate recovery was found to be a major contributing factor in all five patterns of *karoshi*.

RECOVERY: THE VITAL CONCEPT

Recovery is an important word and a vital concept. It means renewal of life and energy. Knowing how and when to recover may prove to be the most important skill in your life.

MORE RECOVERY OR LESS STRESS?

Most traditional stress management programs claim that stress reduction is the best answer for people whose lives are being ground down by stress. The message being pushed is that a high volume of stress is hazardous to health and happiness.

In keeping with that view, the psychological community has been nearly unanimous in recognizing the importance of stress reduction strategies. The underlying assumption is that by reducing stress, one can improve the quality of one's life.

Toughness Training, however, asserts that not the volume of stress alone but rather *the volume of stress relative to the volume of recovery* is the critical factor. As Japan's Institute of Health discovered in each of the five causes of *karoshi,* insufficient recovery relative to the high volume of stress is what kills.

Chapter 3 showed that high stress can weaken you, maintain you, or strengthen you. What high stress does to you depends not on the volume of stress but on how well recovery balances that high stress.

In other words, moderate stress can be balanced by moderate

recovery, but high stress must be balanced by high recovery. We've all heard about high stress for years, but high recovery? Not a familiar concept. It should be, though—either high recovery balances high stress, or *karoshi* does. Take your pick.

And on the most realistic level known to humankind—the choice between life and death—you will take your pick whether you want to or not. It's an unavoidable decision. You can make it deliberately after doing a risk/benefit analysis, or by default as most high-stressed people do. If you're under high stress now that will probably continue, either you balance it with high recovery, or your name goes down in Mr. Karoshi's little black book of early appointments.

If concern about *karoshi* seems too negative a reason to opt for high recovery, here's a more positive one: A high volume of stress is necessary to maintain a high level of toughness. Our goal, then, is not necessarily to reduce stress, but to increase the volume and effectiveness of recovery to a level that balances the stress we face.

RECOVERY IN PHYSICAL TRAINING
AND IN LIFE

Much of what I understand about the importance of recovery in life evolved initially from a 2½-year study of how top professional tennis players managed stress during competition. I wanted to identify the acquired habits of thinking and acting that helped mentally tough competitors manage stress so effectively.

I was convinced that if I looked closely enough, I could isolate the elements of mental toughness. However, months of intense study and analysis revealed few significant differences between the thoughts or actions of top competitors and poor competitors while the ball was in play. This came as a surprise, to say the least.

Not until I began a rigorous study of between-point time did I discover dramatic differences. I soon saw that top competitors and poor competitors thought and acted very differently between points.

The concept of performing between points had never been a serious training consideration. The primary focus of coaches and players had always been on performing during points. The 25 seconds allowed between points had always been viewed simply as the necessary time for players to get to the appropriate place on the court and resume play. From a training perspective, between-point time had always been perceived as unimportant.

Many players and coaches were shocked to learn that as much as 85 percent of a tennis match is between-point time. In a two-hour match the amount of time spent actually playing points can be less than 20 minutes. This realization alone suggested that between-point time plays a far greater part in determining the outcome than most of the tennis world had imagined.

Yet the real breakthrough for me came when I finally grasped that for top competitors, between-point time was *trained recovery.* These competitors had learned to use that time to their fullest competitive advantage, primarily to recover from the stress of the previous point. They also used those precious seconds to put themselves into their best emotional and mental state to win the next point—that is, into their Ideal Performance State.

Compared to poor competitors, top competitors walked differently, carried their head and shoulders differently, breathed differently, and even carried their racquets differently. They also controlled their thoughts and emotions differently. Remote microphones and video replay clearly indicated that top competitors are much more skillful at not allowing negative thoughts and emotions to intrude into the recovery period. Intuitively they had sensed a strong connection linking what they did between points to how they performed during points.

I discovered a remarkable similarity among top competitors in the sequences of their thoughts and actions between points. The same movements, gestures, habits, and rituals kept reappearing. Outwardly, it seemed as if they had all been trained in the same way and were following the same system.

Yet none of the top competitors I studied had been taught about between-point recovery. What they were doing was the result of many years of competition. They had simply learned the most effective way to balance the great physical and emotional stress of competition.

All the data indicated that tough competitors, unlike nontough ones, maximized their opportunities for recovery between points.

They had acquired a highly refined and precise system of trained recovery.

In contrast, poor competitors were less disciplined, less exact, less ritualistic, and more varied in their actions between points. They also were much more likely to express negative emotion each time they made a mistake. When angry, frustrated, disappointed, irritated, or discouraged, they were far more likely to show it.

Not surprisingly, however, as heart rate data invariably indicated, those who outwardly expressed negative emotion and were less disciplined between points experienced more recovery problems. And as heart rates became more linear, indicating that recovery was failing, competitors' play steadily declined. Without the consistent troughs of recovery between points, players eventually lost their ability to expend energy and sustain the competitive fight.

Over and over, the same patterns surfaced. When performing well, players' heart rates were wavelike, not linear. Waves of stress were followed by symmetrical waves of recovery. On the other hand, performance problems closely followed linear heart rates.

Once I understood the importance of between-point recovery time and precisely how top competitors recovered, I began teaching less effective competitors to recover in the same way that top players do. I acted on my hunch that this would result in significant gains in competitive toughness. And that's exactly what happened.

Players quickly learned how to recover better, and by so doing became tougher competitors who won more matches. Over the past few years I've helped merge trained recovery into the daily workouts of coaches and players all over the world. For most, this has led to significant gains in mental toughness and playing success.

Making the vital connection between mental toughness and recovery in tennis was exciting and promising. However, the most stimulating aspect of this discovery lay in another direction entirely. In time I recognized that the playing/nonplaying alternation in tennis provides a powerful example of stress and recovery's dynamic interaction in every area of human activity.

The wavelike action of stress and recovery in tennis parallels that of life in many ways. The during-point time in life is stress/work, and the between-point time is recovery/nonwork. And, just as in tennis, the nonwork time can be used either to prolong cycles of stress and linearity or to induce the waves of recovery that give relief from stress.

Also, in life as in tennis, what has traditionally been viewed as unimportant—and even disgraceful—nonwork time is actually of critical value for balancing stress and recovery. The concept of trained recovery in tennis applies equally well to life. Better, more precise, and stronger recovery in life means greater capacity for energy expenditure.

Consider George, Larry, and Steve, three men who work in the same insurance company office as underwriters. George hangs around the water cooler so much he's in danger of getting fired for it. Larry never goes near the water cooler except once each morning to fill his water bottle so he can satisfy his thirst sitting at his desk. Steve walks over to the water cooler every hour or so, and takes a moment to rib George, or briefly joke around with anyone else who happens to be there.

Although their boss is puzzled by Steve's frequent trips to the cooler, he wisely lets it ride. Steve does more work and makes fewer mistakes than the other two underwriters.

George is a typical case of undertraining. Because he avoids work stress as much as he can, his work capability is declining steadily. At the same time his emotional stress is increasing, because he knows he'll get fired if he doesn't shape up.

Larry, a typical case of overtraining, has the opposite problem. He works all day as hard as he can go, never letting up for a moment. As a result, Larry's continuously overstressed brain makes many mistakes. These take time to rectify, further increasing his stress. By the end of the day Larry is always exhausted, and quick to snarl at anyone who comes near.

Steve works with intense concentration for short periods of time, and then bounces up and forgets his work before sitting down again with a refreshed, recovered mind. He never stays away from his desk long, since he learned early in his career that being away more than a few minutes was counterproductive. At quitting time Steve usually feels relaxed, cheerful, and energetic. That's just one of his rewards for understanding how to oscillate between high stress and a high level of recovery within the limits of his work environment.

It's not hard to predict what will happen to these three men:

George will get fired, Larry will get ulcers, and Steve will get promoted.

Productivity in life depends on one's ability to spike periods of stress and trough periods of recovery. As in sport, fulfillment and achievement in life have firm links to the learned capacity to repeatedly follow periods of heavy energy expenditure with equally significant waves of recovery, followed again by powerful energy expenditure.

The significance of the common saying "Give me a break" goes far beyond its usual use as a throwaway line. A genuine break (as opposed to a phony break—a working lunch, for example) provides temporary relief from linear stress. As we'll come to see in later chapters, we can vastly improve the effectiveness of life's breaks through training.

THE MOST IMPORTANT UNDERSTANDING:

TRAINED RECOVERY IS THE FOUNDATION OF TOUGHNESS BOTH IN LIFE

AND IN SPORT. IF YOU WANT TO GET TOUGHER,

THE REQUIREMENTS ARE FEW AND SIMPLE:

LEARN HOW TO MAKE POWERFUL WAVES OF RECOVERY

AS WELL AS POWERFUL WAVES OF STRESS.

USING NATURE'S RHYTHMS
INSTEAD OF FIGHTING THEM

Rhythm is one of nature's fundamental constants. Living things pulsate, and linearity (the absence of pulsation) is dysfunctional; one need only look about in nature to verify that fact. Earth's daily rhythms of darkness and light influence our biological clocks in pervasive, multiple ways. Energy, alertness, emotional states, muscle strength, and even the immune system's functions show predictable rhythms throughout each day.

Captured in each of the nearly 25,000 breaths we take every 24 hours is the symmetry of stress and recovery in perfect balance. Inhaling is stress, exhaling is recovery. In an average lifetime, each of us will experience over 500,000,000 stress and recovery cycles as we breathe. Inhaling oxygen brings energy; exhaling carbon dioxide brings recovery—and our last breath will bring total linearity. In a real sense, the rhythm of breath reflects the rhythm of all nature.

The nearly 90,000 daily heartbeats are an equally good example of stress and recovery. The hundreds of thousands of stress and recovery cycles pulsating within the brain in the form of EEG activity also reflect life's basic rhythms.

Psychobiology researcher Ernest Rossi has studied our natural rhythms. The cycles of stress and recovery those rhythms create, he contends, work continuously on our minds and bodies in powerful ways. These naturally occurring peaks and troughs, known as Basic Rest-Activity Cycles (BRAC), interact with essential mind-body systems. They affect mood, appetite, sleep, alertness, energy, and performance in the short term and health, wealth, and longevity in the long term.

Biological rhythms called ultradians pulse through us every 90 to 120 minutes; circadians pulse every 24 hours. Rossi believes that continuously overriding the body's naturally occurring ultradian and circadian cycles of stress and rest can lead to a host of serious physical and emotional problems.

These problems include everything from chronic fatigue to weakening the immune system, and from depression to poor performance. A wide range of stress-related research supports Rossi's position. One of these studies shows that workers whose jobs require sustained vigilance over long periods of time without breaks are far more prone to stress-related diseases of all kinds.

Ultradian and circadian researchers refer to the habit of ignoring the body's need for rest and recovery as endurance stress. Breaking cycles of stress every 90 to 120 minutes with 15 to 20 minutes of recovery fits the body's natural needs best, Rossi reports. According to Rossi, these 15- to 20-minute rest breaks restore proper ultradian rhythms and, in so doing, are critical to physical and psychological rejuvenation and long-term health.

Rossi contends that disregarding the body's basic need for recovery depletes the hormonal messenger molecules. This depletion reduces the body's ability to adapt. Glucose and insulin, the messenger molecules that regulate energy—plus the messengers that regulate stress, cortisol and adrenaline—appear to follow ultradian patterns. This further supports Rossi's position.

To Rossi, accident-proneness, bad decision-making, mistakes of omission, and impatience are early signs of poor restoration (recovery). Problems with sleep, heart, immune system, and gastrointestinal function are symptoms of chronic failure to respond to the body's recovery needs.

It's significant that a far larger proportion of serious human accidents—including a high rate of auto smashups—takes place during the early-morning hours than the 24-hour averages would predict. The catastrophic nuclear accidents at Chernobyl and Three Mile Island and the tragic explosion at the Union Carbide plant in Bhopal, India, occurred during the early morning. These events strongly suggest that our circadian rhythms make us vulnerable during the early-morning hours.

THE HIERARCHY OF RECOVERY NEEDS

Two significant issues regarding recovery are establishing which forms of recovery are most important, and understanding how recovery is related to need fulfillment. Abraham Maslow's Hierarchy of Needs, one of the best-known and most practical theories of motivation, is helpful here.

Maslow contended that people satisfy their needs according to a natural system of body and mind priorities. He divided these priorities into deficiency needs and growth needs.

Deficiency needs include life's basic urges: hunger, thirst, and safety. According to Maslow, these have the highest priority. Growth needs include love, self-esteem, and self-actualization. According to Maslow, basic deficiency needs must be satisfied before growth needs.

In other words, the need for food and water is more urgent and has a higher priority than the need for love or self-esteem. Taking this a step further, efforts to satisfy one's need for love and self-esteem will be only weakly felt—and generally left unpursued—until needs for food, water, and safety have been met.

Applying Maslow's Hierarchy of Needs to recovery answered

many questions. The notion that recovery and need fulfillment follow a similar hierarchy made great practical and intuitive sense.

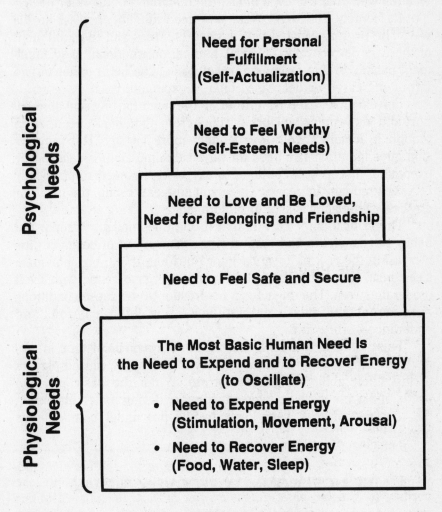

Figure 4.1   Hierarchy of Recovery Needs*

As seen in Figure 4.1, the most basic human need in the context of Toughness Training is to expend and recover energy. The most important forms of stress involve stimulating and moving the

* Adapted from Maslow's *Hierarchy of Needs,* 1962.

physical body; the most important forms of recovery involve eating, drinking, and sleeping. Failure to meet those basic body needs interferes with, and can even block, the fulfillment of all other needs.

Put simply, stress/recovery and need fulfillment relate in this way: The urge associated with a need is stress and the fulfillment of the urge is recovery. Physical, mental, or emotional need fulfillment usually brings feelings of relief. Relief can be in either of two forms: increased or decreased energy expenditure.

For example, exercising to fulfill the need for physical stimulation and movement will bring relief from that basic need, even though it actually involves expending more energy. The progression goes like this: The need for physical stimulation is relieved by exercising, but as you continue to exercise, the need to physically recover gradually increases. Once you stop exercising, the need for physical stimulation starts to build again.

The critical point here is that if one does not meet important bodily needs, stress and recovery are thrown out of balance, thus increasing the risk of linearity. Poor nutrition, thirst, or inadequate sleep beat down our ability to expend energy or cope with even moderate stress. The impact can be drastic. Under these conditions our mental and physical toughness—our fight, passion, and endurance—erode away.

This was clearly evident during the between-point time in tennis. Problems of poor hydration or low blood sugar caused players to lose their ability to tolerate stress. When the basic physical needs of players were no longer being met during match play, even the toughest players were likely to collapse under competition's pressures.

THE MOST COMMON RECOVERY SIGNALS

Since recovery plays such a central role in the toughening process, understanding the signals of recovery is essential in the same way that we found it vital to understand the signals of overtraining and undertraining. The distinction between undertraining and recovery is important here.

As discussed in Chapter 3, undertraining results from insufficient stress and leads to weakening. Recovery, on the other hand, is temporary relief from stress and is essential to toughening. However, linear recovery (too much rest) can result in the weakening condition of undertraining.

PHYSICAL RECOVERY

The most common sign of physical recovery is the feeling of bodily relief. If you've been standing or walking for a long time, sitting down brings immediate muscular relief. In contrast, if you've been sitting on an airplane or stuck behind your desk for hours, getting up and moving around will also bring muscular relief. This example shows that physical relief can occur when levels of physical activity either increase or decrease. However, the most common situation is for physical relief to come from reduced physical activity.

THE IMPORTANCE OF RECOGNIZING
HOW PHYSICAL RECOVERY FEELS

Increasing one's awareness of how physical recovery actually feels is extremely important in recovery training. In addition to the feeling of relief that comes with satisfying hunger, thirst, or sleepiness, the most common signals of physical recovery are the bodily sensations associated with decreases in heart rate, breath rate, blood pressure, muscle tension, and brain activity. As heart rate decreases, as breathing becomes slower and deeper, as blood pressure drops, the process of physical recovery begins.

The first critical step in recovery training is to learn to recognize when physical recovery is occurring and how it feels. Tuning in to decreasing muscle tension in your hands or neck, feeling the relaxation of your chest muscles as you breathe more deeply, is listening to the language of physical recovery.

THE MOST COMMON SIGNS OF PHYSICAL RECOVERY

- Feelings of bodily relief (reduced feelings of hunger, thirst, sleepiness, tension, and so forth)
- Decreasing heart rate (reduced electrocardiographic, or EKG, activity)

- Decreasing breath rate (decreased respiratory activity)
- Decreasing blood pressure
- Decreasing muscle tension (reduced electromyographic, or EMG, activity)
- Decreasing blood cortisone (the primary stress hormone)
- Decreasing oxygen consumption
- Decreasing electrical brain waves (reduced electroencephalographic, or EEG, activity—from beta to alpha, theta, or delta frequencies)
- Increasing electrical skin resistance, or ESR (As relaxation increases, the rate of perspiration decreases, causing skin resistance to increase and "skin talk" to decrease.)

EMOTIONAL RECOVERY

Emotional stress takes many forms, from gut-wrenching pain to subtle, nondescript feelings of anxiety, pressure, and uneasiness. The most common sign of emotional recovery is the feeling that at least for the moment, there is a break in the emotional storm.

Relief from fear, guilt, anger, depression, or doubt signals movement toward recovery. Relief means a lifted spirit, a happier, healthier, more positive outlook and attitude. An increase in positive feelings such as fun, joy, humor, and happiness and a decrease in negative feelings indicate that a wave of recovery has begun.

The shift from negative to positive feelings signals the onset of recovery waves that may be brief and weak or prolonged and powerful. Whether they are weak or powerful, the important issue is that the emotional shift represents movement away from stress and toward recovery.

Once basic physiological needs for food, water, and rest have been met, recovery from emotional needs associated with physical safety and psychological security have the greatest urgency and power. Most anxiety and pressure in people's lives stem from perceived threats associated with psychological security issues. Relief from needs for love, self-esteem, and personal fulfillment become increasingly more important and pressing as safety and security needs are met. Within that context, feelings of increased love and self-esteem usually signal powerful emotional recovery.

──────── **THE MOST COMMON SIGNS OF EMOTIONAL RECOVERY** ────────

- A feeling of emotional relief
- Increasing positive feelings—fun, joy, humor, happiness
- Decreasing negative feelings of anger, frustration, and bitterness
- Increasing feelings of safety and security
- Decreasing feelings of depression, sadness, guilt, or grief
- Decreasing feelings of pressure
- Increasing feelings of being loved
- Increasing feelings of self-esteem
- Increasing feelings of personal fulfillment

MENTAL RECOVERY

Intense mental activity—such as preparing a difficult financial report, analyzing a challenging technical paper, or studying a complex subject—can be very stressful. This is true even when the person doing the mental work feels no emotional stress about the activity whatsoever. All by itself, intense mental work takes a significant amount of energy. In other words, mental work can be very stressful.

Relief from mental stress can take many forms. Allowing one's mind to drift away to some faraway place, to fantasize about going fishing, taking a nap, or vacationing, brings momentary relief.

Such a fleeting moment of fantasy produces only a small wave of recovery. However, a walk around the block or a ten-minute nutrition break often will produce a significant recovery wave.

Mental recovery is generally associated with increased feelings of calmness and a general sense that things are slowing down mentally. As mental stress decreases, mental focus tends to broaden and become more diffuse. A narrow, precise mental focus indicates continuing stress. Mental recovery is associated with an increase in fantasy, creativity, and imagery. As these qualities increase, the feelings of mental relief usually follow suit.

- Feeling of relief mentally
- Increasing calmness (reduced EEG activity)
- Increasing sense of slowing down mentally (reduced EEG activity)
- Broadening of mental focus (as stress increases, mental focus narrows)
- Increasing fantasy
- Increasing creativity
- Increasing detachment
- Increasing imagery

TRAINING TO SLEEP, EAT, AND REST MORE EFFECTIVELY

Tennis allows a maximum of only 25 seconds between points for recovery. For poor competitors, that simply isn't enough time to get ready to play the next point. Their undisciplined, unstructured approach to the 25-second recovery opportunity simply fails time after time.

The story is very different for top competitors. By resting their eyes on the strings of their racquets to control arousal and avoid distraction, by regulating the depth and rhythm of their breathing, and by controlling their actions and thoughts during the 25 seconds, they make the stress of the previous point manageable.

Their competitive success is clearly tied to taking full advantage of each opportunity for rest and recovery. Their ability to wrest maximum recovery from those brief intervals plays an essential part in sharpening their competitive edge.

Although not as frequent or clearly defined as in tennis, recovery opportunities in life certainly exist. If a tennis player can compress recovery into intervals of 25 seconds, imagine what could be done with 5-, 10-, or 15-minute breaks if we train for recovery as they do.

How much better would we manage our job-related stress if we phased out our unstructured, sedentary coffee breaks and trained and organized ourselves to take powerful recovery breaks? We could keep things interesting by rotating exercise breaks, laugh breaks, breathing breaks, and nutrition breaks. To answer the question, we would manage our present job-related stress vastly better, and soon be looking for more opportunities.

How much more stress could be balanced if we considered the hours away from work as opportunities for trained recovery? For ourselves and for our loved ones, learning how to train recovery may be one of the most important life skills that we'll ever acquire.

Put simply, trained recovery is learning how to get the maximum recovery benefit from sleeping, eating, and freedom from work stress. The sheer volume of stress in most people's lives today cannot be sufficiently balanced with a casual, nonspecific approach to recovery. A sound recovery base is the first priority in Toughness Training.

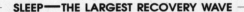

SLEEP—THE LARGEST RECOVERY WAVE

Apart from breathing, satisfying thirst, and eating, sleep clearly is the most important recovery activity in our lives. It's also the

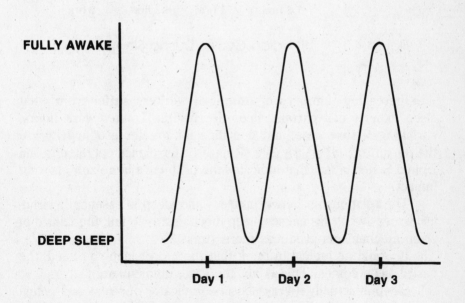

Figure 4.2   Normal Wake/Sleep Cycles

body's largest circadian rhythm. Disruptions of this critical recovery rhythm can have serious health and performance consequences.

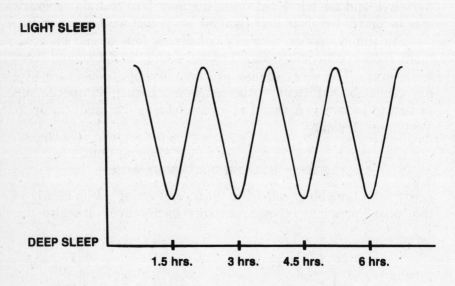

LIGHT SLEEP

DEEP SLEEP

1.5 hrs.   3 hrs.   4.5 hrs.   6 hrs.

Figure 4.3   Ultradian Cycles During Sleep

Increasing numbers of American workers suffer from what sleep experts call chronic sleep deprivation. Longer work hours, shrinking leisure time, and demands for greater productivity are the norm. In 1991 nearly 200 sleep disorder clinics operated in the United States, a fact that indicates the problem's large and growing impact.

The relationship between stress and sleep is essentially circular. Excessive stress causes sleep mechanisms to fail; the failure of sleep mechanisms produces more stress.

It would be logical to think that the more sleep you need, the easier sleep comes. This is not the case, unfortunately.

Sleep is actually a very sensitive indicator of stress and recovery balance. Ironically, excessive stress often blocks the very thing needed most.

Just how much sleep one requires depends on the individual and the current volume of stress. Many sleep studies have been made that isolate people for weeks from all time cues, alarms, or clocks. These studies show that under normal stress conditions, people naturally sleep about one-third of the time—about 8 hours out of every 24.

During that eight-hour recovery phase of sleeping, researchers have discovered that individuals pass through four to six distinct ultradian cycles of sleep every 90 to 120 minutes. Each cycle has five stages.

Stages One and Two are periods of light sleep during which muscles relax, body temperature and blood pressure fall, and brain waves pulse between four and eight cycles per second. This type of sleep consumes nearly half of one's total sleeping time.

Stages Three and Four are periods of deep sleep. Here metabolic rate and muscle tension reach their lowest levels, and brain waves decline to less than four cycles per second. Sleep researchers have linked feeling deeply rested upon awakening with successful entry into Stages Three and Four of the sleep cycle.

Stage Five is called REM (Rapid Eye Movement) sleep. Breathing quickens, blood pressure and heart rate become irregular, and brain waves accelerate to 13 to 35 cycles per second. Most dreaming occurs during REM.

TAKE UNLAZY NAPS

Of further interest in the context of recovery and sleep is the urge to nap. Although often thought of as a sign of laziness, the desire for an afternoon nap is actually a natural biological rhythm. According to sleep researchers, the need to sleep typically occurs twice within a 24-hour cycle.

The first circadian trough coincides with darkness and is strong and prolonged. The second occurs in middle to late afternoon; its strength depends on the volume and depth of sleep the previous night. An afternoon nap as short as ten minutes can provide substantial physiological and psychological recovery, particularly if it is synchronized to the body's natural urge to rest. Increased energy, concentration, alertness, and motivation have been associated with afternoon naps. Current data suggest that naps generally should not last longer than ninety minutes. Awakening from a nap feeling groggy and tired usually indicates a continuing sleep deficiency.

<hr>

HOW SLEEP CYCLES GET OFF TRACK

Yowling cats, midnight earthquakes, and early-morning phone calls usually have only a temporary effect. Many other factors affect natural sleep cycles for longer periods.

More people are sensitive to caffeine doesn't bother them or that it's only found in coffee. Not true. Tea, soft drinks, and chocolate all contain enough caffeine to deny sound sleep to people who have become sensitized to this stimulant.

More people are sensitive to caffeine than will admit it, for fear of having to give up a favorite beverage or snack. Anyone who is emotionally tough—or who aspires to be—will have no difficulty choosing a good night's sleep over the momentary pleasure of caffeine intake.

If you're not sleeping as well as you think you should, look for simple solutions first. You can't be sure that caffeine isn't the culprit even if you don't take any after noontime unless you test carefully for it.

It isn't hard. First, identify every source of caffeine in your regular diet, and then make sure you avoid all of it for three days. It can take that long to flush all the residual caffeine out of your system. If you're sensitized to caffeine, it doesn't take much to shatter sleep.

Caffeine works as a stimulant that interferes with several processes contributing to healthy sleep. Sensitivity to it grows slowly over time until it abruptly becomes critical. Many people who in the past could drink their fill of coffee anytime and still get a refreshing night's sleep suddenly can't anymore. Sometimes just a morning wake-up cup or two of coffee—or caffeine-laden soft drinks in the afternoon—can keep them restless long into the night.

Other common sleep enemies include alcohol; irregular sleep hours; the timing of meals; exercise intensity, duration, and timing; the volume of overall stress; and jet lag from crossing time zones.

Alcohol works as a central nervous system depressant to suppress part of REM sleep. This is one reason why "sleeping it off" produces a hangover—the drinker was unconscious without gaining the enormous benefit of REM sleep.

Consistency of sleep hours is an important element in the healthy regulation of sleep. Constantly changing the times of going to bed and getting up is highly disruptive to natural sleep rhythms.

The consumption of large meals just prior to sleep is also disruptive. This is primarily because of the natural stress associated with the digestion of food.

Regular exercise, especially in the late afternoon, promotes overall relaxation and generally enhances sleep, often by easing the impact of emotional stress.

When overall stress is high, particularly if much of it is emotional stress—fear, guilt, dread, frustration, anger, and so on—these negative emotions can overpower the body's natural need for sleep.

Not until the jet age dawned did changing time zones become a commonplace problem. Before then it was difficult to travel quickly enough to disturb the body's natural biological clocks that regulate sleep mechanisms. Now any transcontinental or transoceanic flight will knock them out of kilter.

STABILIZING THE HUNGER/THIRST WAVE

After catching one's breath, consuming adequate amounts of food and water is the recovery with the highest priority. If nutritional and hydration needs are not sufficiently met, all stress becomes excessive and all recovery mechanisms soon fail. Follow these guidelines to stabilize the hunger/thirst recovery mechanism:

- Establish a regular, consistent schedule of eating and drinking.
- Adjust the volume of food and drink to meet the demands for energy expenditure. Professional athletes may require more than 4,000 calories a day, and up to 320 ounces of water when exercising in hot weather. To remain healthy and avoid weight gain, nonexercisers may require as little as 1,500 calories a day and less than 40 ounces of water. Find out what your needs are and take care of them.
- Eat and drink often—every two to three hours if possible. Frequent small meals help to stabilize blood sugar, giving you more energy over longer periods of time. Consume four to five meals

per day, but eat lightly. Breakfast is essential. Unless you put gas in your tank before you start your day, your engine won't deliver full power. Eating lightly means less digestive stress and less hunger. Eating often helps reduce any unhealthy preoccupation with food that might be creeping up on you, and reduces the urge to eat big meals. Your goal throughout the day should be to never feel totally full or totally famished.

- Eat early rather than late in the evening. If you want to be asleep by 11:00, meals after 8:30 are disruptive.
- Whenever possible, avoid putting two important recovery activities back to back, such as eating a big meal and then going directly to bed. As much as you can, organize your routine so that a cycle of energy expenditure follows every important recovery activity.
- Eat as wide a variety of foods as possible with a preference for natural, fresh foods that are free of preservatives and chemical contaminants. Eating a wide diversity of foods gives you the best chance of fulfilling all your nutritional needs.
- Eat low-fat, carbohydrate-rich foods. At least 60 to 70 percent of your daily calories should be derived from carbohydrates, no more than 15 to 20 percent from fat, and 10 to 15 percent from protein.
- Avoid simple sugars. They can spike blood sugar levels, a condition that's often followed by low blood sugar.

HOW POOR RECOVERY UNDERMINES YOU
IN LIFE AND SPORT

If you watch tennis tournaments much, you'll occasionally see a player make great shots in the first two sets and win them decisively. It looks as though he has the match in the bag.

Then he starts missing shots he should have made and goes on to lose the next two sets. In the fifth set he's hopelessly outclassed. It's hard to believe this is the same player who looked so strong in the first part of the match.

It's easy to say that sensing victory after two sets, he choked, lost his concentration, or relaxed—and blew a match he could easily have won. Those things happen, of course, but not as often as many people think. More likely he failed because he started the match inadequately recovered.

Recovered from what?

From physical or psychological stress that could have arisen from any number of sources. He may have been seriously over-trained or undertrained; he may be under some personal emotional stress that kept him from getting adequate rest and nutrition; he may have reached the court too excited to realize that he was close to dehydration or inadequately fed for a long match.

Any of those can cause a player to hit the wall physically. Run out of gas. Die on his feet. When that happens, when we're faced with physical stress but our bodies are dehydrated or out of energy that only food can supply, we all stumble. Our fight melts. Our skills vanish. We lose.

Although this chain of events is most visible in professional sport, it happens vastly more often in ordinary life. Business executives too stressed out to make profitable decisions; salespeople too stressed out to make convincing presentations; parents too stressed out to control their kids—but in every case it wasn't really too much stress that did the damage, it was too little recovery.

KEY POINT:

WITHOUT ENOUGH FOOD, WATER, AND SLEEP, WE ALL

BECOME WIMPS AND LOSE. SUCCESS IN EVERY FIELD

OF HUMAN ENDEAVOR REQUIRES ADEQUATE RECOVERY.

NUTRITIONAL GUIDELINES

EAT AND DRINK MORE:
Fruits
Vegetables, particularly green leafy ones
Salads, pasta, rice, whole-grain breads, oatmeal, cereals that have
   no sugar added
Egg whites, plain yogurt, turkey, and chicken
Meats and vegetables that have been broiled or grilled
Fruit juices and water

EAT AND DRINK LESS:
Fried meat
Red meat no matter how cooked
Fried vegetables
Butter, margarine, mayonnaise
Creamy salad dressings: Ranch, French, Blue Cheese, Thousand Island, Creamy Italian
Egg yolks (the yellow part), ice cream, doughnuts, danishes, cookies, candy
Soft drinks and alcoholic beverages

ACTIVE VERSUS PASSIVE REST

Because recovery from physical, emotional, and mental stress can occur from movement as well as nonmovement of the physical body, the distinction between passive and active rest is important.

Ideal recovery for someone who has been physically active most of the day is nonmovement; for someone who has been sedentary most of the day, it is movement.

As seen previously, active rest involves physical activities that break normal cycles of physical, emotional, and mental stress. Examples include walking, yoga, stretching, and fishing. Sports activities such as jogging, biking, tennis, and golf—if done on a noncompetitive basis—are also excellent. Business executives seeking to recover from the stress of business competition get little benefit from stressful competition at play.

Passive rest involves nonphysical activities that break normal cycles of stress. Examples include meditation, massage, reading, listening to music, deep breathing, and naps.

The distinction between active and passive rest is important to the discussion of recovery strategies that is to follow.

-- ACTIVE REST --

Nonvigorous activities involving physical movement that break normal cycles of physical, emotional, and mental stress are recommended for active rest. Examples:

- Walking
- Yoga
- Stretching
- Tai-chi
- Fishing
- Noncompetitive sport activities such as golf, swimming, hiking, jogging, biking, tennis

-- PASSIVE REST --

Activities that break normal cycles of physical, emotional, and mental stress without involving physical body movement are recommended for passive rest. Examples:

- Meditation
- Watching TV, movies
- Massage
- Deep breathing
- Whirlpool bath
- Afternoon nap
- Reading
- Listening to music

RECOVERY STRATEGIES FOR PHYSICAL (OUTSIDE-IN) STRESS

-- RECOVERY NEEDS STEMMING FROM --
-- INTENSE PHYSICAL ACTIVITY --

The following recovery steps will be helpful after prolonged physical activity:

- Make sure that basic physiological needs for food, water, and sleep are adequately met.
- Get involved in nonphysical activities (passive rest) that decrease muscle activity and tension (reduce EMG activity). Common examples include reading, watching movies or TV, listening to music, deep breathing, massage, meditation, and EMG feedback.

RECOVERY NEEDS STEMMING FROM
PROLONGED PHYSICAL INACTIVITY

The following steps will be helpful for nonexercisers who want to adopt a more active life-style, and for others who have somehow failed to get adequate exercise for a period of years.

- Make certain that basic physiological needs for food, water, and sleep are adequately met.
- Have a physician give you a complete physical examination before beginning your more active regime.
- Get involved in physical activities (active rest) that increase muscle activity and blood flow. Common examples are walking, stretching, biking, sports participation of all kinds, running, swimming, weight lifting, exercise machines, and rebound exercise.
- Ease into your exercise routine slowly if you're overweight, very slowly if you're overweight and over forty.

RECOVERY STRATEGIES FOR EMOTIONAL (INSIDE-OUT) STRESS

RECOVERY NEEDS STEMMING FROM INTENSE EMOTIONAL STRESS

This category also includes situations where the emotional stress has been endured for prolonged periods. In both cases, the following steps will be helpful:

- Make certain that basic physiological needs for food, water, and sleep are adequately met.

- If possible, temporarily remove yourself from all stressors—take a break. Ideally your break to recover from a heavy emotional hit will be a long vacation, or at least a week or a weekend away. Even an overnight stay can often be useful. At the very least, get out of the house and see a film at a theater, preferably one that will trigger strong positive emotions.
- Get involved in some kind of physical exercise (active rest). Physical stress often provides temporary emotional recovery.
- Express your emotions verbally. Be careful, however, not to express negative emotion in a performance situation. Expressing negative feelings and emotions during competition or within the work setting usually undermines performance.
- Express your emotions in writing. Getting painful feelings down on paper often provides temporary emotional recovery—and since it can be done in private, this outlet can be risk-free.
- Get involved in mental or physical activities that decrease brain activity. Common examples are passive rest activities— meditation, deep breathing, listening to music—and active rest activities—yoga, walking, tai-chi, easy biking.
- Use humor and laughter to break the cycle of excessive emotional stress. Humor tapes, video comedies, and people who make you laugh have great value. Laughter quickly reduces the flow of emotional stress hormones. In terms of recovery, laughter is serious business.

EMOTIONAL RECOVERY THROUGH TALKING

The exact neurochemical mechanism is still unclear, but emotionally traumatic events can get stored by the brain so that they are not readily accessible to conscious thought. This seems to occur instinctively to protect the body from an overload of stress hormones that can have serious consequences for the mind and body. Stress hormones powerfully affect nearly every system in the body.

Blocking traumatic events from consciousness acts essentially as a survival and recovery mechanism. This often happens during childhood. Deaths, serious accidents, sexual abuse, and physical abuse are severe stressors that often get stored away from consciousness as a means of protection. The brain's task then is to gradually allow dissipation of the emotionally charged event over time. Brief, sudden flashbacks and mysterious intrusions of painful events long past can occur for years.

Chronic depression is often a consequence of the brain's failure to dissipate emotionally charged memories so that full recovery becomes possible. Although the events are not conscious, they may continue to affect brain chemistry and function and can be seriously disruptive to normal mind and body functions.

Blocking traumatic events from consciousness provides short-term relief from emotional stress. However, this response can lead to chronic repression and block healthy recovery. Such nonspecific psychological pain in the form of persistent depression, unhappiness, confusion, and low self-esteem is often the result of inadequate recovery from past traumatic events.

One of the most effective ways to access such stored information about long-past events to get emotional relief is through talking. Most forms of psychotherapy involve verbally accessing painful memories that have never fully dissipated. Talking is a very important strategy for emotional recovery.

Emotional health is reflected in individuals who have learned to seek and find relief from emotional stress by more direct forms of recovery (talking and writing) than by completely blocking the stressor from consciousness. The more information the brain has to protect from consciousness, the less emotional flexibility and responsiveness is generally shown in stressful situations. Habitually seeking emotional relief through repression leads to a highly rigid, defensive, dysfunctional personality.

RECOVERY NEEDS STEMMING FROM
INSUFFICIENT EMOTIONAL STRESS

This includes lack of sufficient emotional stimulation. In all these cases, the following steps will be helpful:

- Make sure that basic physiological needs for food, water, and sleep are adequately met.
- Get involved in some form of competitive exercise or sport. Rather than simply jogging or hitting tennis balls for exercise, enter races or tournaments. Competition stimulates emotional arousal.

- Get involved in activities that are both physically and emotionally challenging. Activities that have elements of risk or pressure stimulate the greatest arousal. Climb mountains, go snow skiing or skydiving. Take up interpretive dance, or try something else you've never done before that's physically and emotionally challenging.
- Get involved in nonphysical activities that are emotionally challenging. Go back to school and learn a new language or study some intriguing and difficult subject, join Toastmasters and become an effective public speaker, find an amateur theatrical group and act in plays.

RECOVERY STRATEGIES FOR MENTAL (INSIDE-OUT) STRESS

RECOVERY NEEDS STEMMING FROM INTENSE MENTAL STRESS

This includes cases of prolonged or intense thinking, concentrating, computing, and so on.

- Make sure that basic physiological needs for food, water, and sleep are adequately met.
- Involve yourself in physical exercise of some kind. Physical stress breaks the cycle of mental stress almost immediately.
- If possible, take a complete break from mental activity. If that's not feasible, change to a different type of mental activity. For example, change from computing finances to proofreading a manuscript or preparing a speech.
- Get involved in passive rest activities that decrease brain activity.

RECOVERY NEEDS STEMMING FROM INSUFFICIENT MENTAL STRESS

- Make sure that basic physiological needs for food, water, and sleep are adequately met.
- Get involved in areas of new learning, new reading, new listening, and new talking. Search for subjects and activities that are

intellectually challenging, appealing, and fun. Activities that challenge you emotionally often challenge you mentally as well.

OVERVIEW OF RECOMMENDATIONS
FOR TRAINED RECOVERY

- Take a 15- or 20-minute break every 90 to 120 minutes, particularly during periods of high physical, mental, or emotional stress.
- Learn to take naps easily and quickly without feeling groggy or tired afterward.
- During periods of high stress, take an afternoon nap of 10 minutes to an hour whenever possible.
- Get a minimum of 7 to 8 hours of sleep every 24 hours. Carefully monitor sleep activities during periods of high stress.
- If possible, establish a sleep cycle of going to bed early, between 10:00 and midnight, and getting up early, between 6:00 and 8:00 in the morning.
- Go to bed and get up within half an hour of your normal resting cycle every day.
- Keep a daily record of the quantity and quality of sleep, particularly during periods of high stress.
- Eat light, healthful meals according to a regular schedule.
- Always have a nourishing breakfast.
- Consume some form of carbohydrates every two hours, particularly during periods of high stress.
- Drink a minimum of four to six glasses of water per day.
- Avoid putting two significant recovery periods back to back—or two periods of heavy energy expenditure back to back.
- Use daily exercise to break the cycle of high emotional or high mental stress.
- If possible, exercise in the late afternoon.
- In addition to engaging in physical exercise, learn and use at least two specific recovery strategies that provide effective relief for your typical kind of stress. For example, choose yoga, deep breathing, meditation, or keeping a daily diary of your feelings about your world.
- Become very skillful at recognizing your own signs of physical,

emotional, and mental stress as well as those of physical, emotional, and mental recovery.

- Become very skillful at maximizing opportunities for active and passive rest throughout the day. During periods of high stress, make as many waves of recovery as possible throughout the day.
- Monitor your sense of fun and enjoyment daily. Fun is the best single barometer of your recovery strategy's effectiveness, and often of the recovery itself. Fun generally indicates a healthy relationship between stress and recovery. When you're having fun, you're literally recovering emotional energy.

FUN VS. HARD WORK AND DISCIPLINE

Most of us understand the value of hard work and discipline, but we must also realize the value of making work fun. To the extent that we can work hard and maintain a climate of enjoyment and fun, we decrease the volume of emotional and mental stress and the risk of overtraining. Remember, having fun is essentially a state of mind, and as such is highly controllable.

THE MOST IMPORTANT AND BENEFICIAL FORMS OF RECOVERY

- Achieve relief from excessive stress (linearity) through regular cycles of exercise, sleep, episodes of active and passive rest, laughter, and fun.
- Achieve relief from the need for stimulation and arousal (linearity) through exercise and emotional risk-taking.
- Achieve relief from the need for sleep by adhering to well-defined sleep rituals and midafternoon naps.
- Achieve relief from emotional needs on a short-term basis through exercise and on a long-term basis through talking and writing about your feelings and by establishing close healthy friendships.
- Achieve relief from hunger by consuming nutritionally rich foods.

- Achieve relief from hunger by eating often and lightly, and by consuming foods that are high in fiber and carbohydrates.

THE MOST DESTRUCTIVE AND LEAST BENEFICIAL FORMS OF RECOVERY

- Achieve relief from excessive stress (linearity) by abusing alcohol or using drugs such as tranquilizers, marijuana, and so on.
- Achieve relief from the need for stimulation and arousal (linearity) through drugs such as caffeine, amphetamines, and cocaine.
- Achieve relief from the need for sleep through taking drugs that either induce sleep or override the body's demand for sleep.
- Achieve momentary relief from stress by smoking cigarettes.
- Achieve momentary relief from emotional needs by consuming unneeded food.
- Achieve relief from hunger by consuming nutritionally poor foods.
- Achieve relief from emotional stress by habitually oversleeping.

SUMMARY

The urge to eat, drink, sleep, relax, and exercise is the special language of recovery; it represents a window into the physiology of your body. Learning to hear and understand this language is hearing the rhythms and pulsations of life itself.

Our bodies are constantly talking, constantly reaching our conscious minds—or failing to make the connection because the way is blocked by alcohol, drugs, emotion, or a fixed decision to ignore the messages. When the volume of stress in our lives threatens to overwhelm us, we often fail to heed, or even hear, our body's cries for recovery.

We also often fail to recognize that opportunities for recovery are everywhere. To be stronger and tougher we must train to understand and utilize our opportunities for recovery, just as the most successful tennis players use the between-point time.

Tending to our body's need for physiological recovery should always be our first priority. Unfortunately, as we become increasingly more stressed, we neglect the body's basic needs for food, sleep, exercise, and relaxation.

The cost of these many vital neglects is often very high in terms of health, happiness, and productivity. The cost for all too many of us is our most precious possession—the years of healthy life that remain.

Recovery is serious business not just for professional tennis players—it's critically important to us all.

5

CYCLING THROUGH

ROUGH TIMES

No matter where you are on the scale of rough times at the moment, sooner or later even rougher times are going to slam into your life.

Crisis and adversity are deeply woven into the fabric of human existence. Crime, accident, divorce, unemployment, illness, war, addiction, betrayal, a loved one's death, cash-flow problems—the list goes on and on. Directly or indirectly, calamities and tragedies touch us all. Sometimes they strike like sledgehammers.

What are we to do when we take a direct emotional hit, when an unexpected life crisis rocks our soul? How can we continue moving forward with our lives and minimize the damage to our health and psyches?

SURVIVAL TACTICS

Before analyzing four real case studies, let's first establish a few fundamental guidelines for handling rough times. Here are nine survival basics:

1. TRAIN EVERY DAY TO GET AS TOUGH AS POSSIBLE PHYSICALLY AND EMOTIONALLY.
Do this to elevate your health, boost your productivity, and expand your happiness—and for one other vital reason: so that you will suffer less devastation when you absorb your next emotional hit.

Many people think Benjamin Franklin felt pessimistic when he said, "Nothing is certain except death and taxes." Actually he spoke optimistically in ignoring the third category of inevitable events: the emotional blows we all must accept as part of the price of living.

Chances are you have already suffered some hard emotional knocks. You may feel you've paid your dues in this regard. Sadly, it doesn't work that way. More emotional pain will come into your life—and mine too. The only question is when.

A major life crisis is simply a massive dose of stress. If your range of coping is quite limited, a sudden life crisis can swiftly push you beyond your limits into the gray zone where people do destructive things to themselves. That's why it's important to always consider yourself in training to get physically and emotionally stronger.

Keep in mind that the question is never if rough times will come, but simply when and what they will be. In a real sense, every day of our lives represents another opportunity to get tougher and to expand our capacity for coping. I urge you to put this concept to work for you: "Give me stress, I need the practice."

2. HAVE YOUR RECOVERY STRATEGIES TRAINED AND READY.
Stress won't break you, but failing to create sufficient waves of recovery can. High linear stress is lethal, but high stress with relief not only is manageable but can actually be used to get tougher and stronger.

A sudden, massive dose of stress requires an equivalent volume of intense recovery; unless you get the required recovery the stress will eventually beat you down by exceeding your adaptation threshold.

3. DURING TIMES OF HIGH STRESS, DON'T RELY ON THE BODY'S NATURAL RECOVERY URGES.

Expect the natural urges to lose emotional impact under conditions of excessive stress. This means you must make yourself eat, drink, sleep, exercise, and rest according to your regular schedule whether you feel those needs or not. In rough times the safest thing to rely on is an established routine.

4. ATTRIBUTE SOME POSITIVE MEANING TO THE TRAGEDY OR LIFE CRISIS.

Try to see the stressful event as serving some useful purpose such as reestablishing important values in your life, deepening personal relationships, strengthening religious or spiritual beliefs, or building needed toughness. Giving meaning and personal significance to a crisis immediately reduces the destructive power of the negative stressor.

5. LISTEN CAREFULLY TO THE SIGNALS OF EXCESSIVE STRESS.

Feelings of helplessness, fatigue, depression, confusion, doubt, self-blame, and similar agonies are common during times of great crisis. Expect to have such negative feelings after taking a heavy hit; although painful, they are normal in the immediate aftermath of rough times. However, if they persist for a long time, negative feelings of the kinds mentioned strongly indicate a serious need for increased emotional recovery.

6. RELY HEAVILY ON EXERCISE AND TALKING DURING TIMES OF GREAT CRISIS.

Exercising and talking are two of the most powerful and readily available forms of emotional recovery discovered thus far. Forms of active rest, which involve movement of the physical body, and verbally expressing one's feelings with loved ones provide great emotional relief for most people.

7. TAKE CARE OF THE BODY'S BASIC PHYSIOLOGICAL NEEDS FIRST.

Although emotional recovery is clearly the strongest felt need, the basic requirements for food, water, sleep, and relaxation continue to remain highest on the priority list. Nonfulfillment of these silent needs completely undermines the body's capacity for coping.

8. AVOID USING ALCOHOL OR DRUGS TO ACCELERATE RECOVERY PROCESSES DURING CRISES.

Tranquilizers, mood elevators, antidepressants, and sleep medications are often prescribed by physicians, especially for patients who demand instant relief. However, the substantial risk of side effects and of acquiring a chemical dependency means that using such drugs should be considered a recovery strategy of last resort.

9. LOOK FOR SOME SLIVER OF SMOOTHNESS IN EVEN THE ROUGHEST OF TIMES.

Regardless of the blows life pounds you with, you will survive. After all, there's no good alternative. With determination you can tough it out and go on to a better future.

Once you have those ideas firmly in mind, it's easier to look on life's body blows as exercises in damage control. A traumatic life crisis can either strengthen or weaken you. The outcome will turn on (1) how effectively you structure recovery opportunities on a regular, systematic basis during the crisis, (2) how successful you are in making the crisis meaningful in your life—not simply a cruel act of fate, and (3) your acquired level of toughness..

CASE STUDIES

DEATH OF A LOVED ONE

Rita is 53 years old. Her husband, John, died of a heart attack at age 58. Rita and John had been very happily married for 27 years. She has two surviving children, ages 24 and 25. Rita doesn't work. Savings and her husband's life insurance are adequate for her financial needs. Completely devastated emotionally, Rita can't imagine going forward with her life.

Fortunately, she has a good network of friends, and one of her daughters lives only 20 minutes from her home. A deeply religious person, Rita reports an overwhelming sense of loss and depression. She says she cries constantly, and feels that she's "breaking into pieces inside." Most of the time Rita believes she "can't go on alone." She often says, "The house is cold and empty without him."

In addition to her intense grief, Rita has not been able to sleep well since the tragedy. She has also lost her appetite and says, "I don't feel like cooking just for me." When alone, Rita eats only bread and cold cuts, and she never has breakfast. Consequently, Rita has lost 12 pounds and, according to her doctor, was already 5 pounds underweight before her husband died.

Although Rita's primary emotion is one of grief and loss, she also reports that at times she feels angry, bitter, and extremely negative. In addition, she has periods when she feels guilty about her husband's death, as if there were something she could have done to prevent it.

Toughness Training Interventions

The first step, a very important one, calls for organizing a carefully planned, well-structured daily schedule. The purpose is to ensure that Rita's basic needs for food, water, sleep, and exercise are met.

Adhering to a precise schedule during periods of extreme crisis reestablishes a sense of control and order in one's life. Simply doing what you feel like doing at the moment all too often means doing nothing—what you really feel is depression, helplessness, and total disinterest. Without a schedule that forces them to repeatedly create waves of stress and recovery throughout the day, grief-stricken people often shut down, and become dangerously linear.

The best person to create and encourage Rita to follow the daily schedule is Rita's daughter. Together they plan every hour of every day for seven days at a time. Sunday afternoons are used to review the previous week's schedule and prepare the routine for the next seven days.

Here is Rita's recommended schedule for the first seven days following the funeral:

6:30 A.M.   Rita gets up and dresses for 7:00 Mass. The goal here is to regulate Rita's sleep so that she awakens early and retires early. Going to church, an activity she finds deeply satisfying, gives her the incentive to get her day going. The trip out represents a mild form of physical stress; being in church and praying represents emotional recovery.

6:50   Picked up by her daughter, Jill.

7:00–7:30   Mass. Rita's religious beliefs help provide meaning and acceptance of her husband's death. This is a very critical factor in controlling the volume of stress.

7:30–8:15   Rita and Jill have breakfast together. This ensures that Rita will eat breakfast; Jill can observe what she eats and encourage her to eat properly.

8:20   Jill drops Rita off at home.

8:30–9:30   Work for only one hour each day, storing and putting away John's things. Emotionally, this is very painful, but Rita insists on doing it alone. Although highly stressful, this period is an important grieving time for Rita that has considerable long-term value. This is limited, however, to one hour a day because of the intense emotional anguish it triggers.

9:30–10:00   A 30-minute walk around the neighborhood. The active rest cycle is particularly important at this time because of the stressful nature of the previous hour.

10:00–10:15   Light carbohydrate recovery snack. Fruit or natural juice will help stabilize blood sugar levels and maintain energy.

10:15–11:30   Scheduled visits by friends to her house or talks on the phone with them. Although Rita occasionally cries and becomes highly emotional during this time, talking plays a vital part in full and healthy recovery.

11:30–12:00   Read Bible and pray. This is a satisfying time for Rita. She reports a great sense of peace and relief during this 30-minute period.

12:00–12:15 P.M.   Preparation of lunch for herself and daughter. Jill has been able to adjust her schedule so she can take a two-hour lunch break. This enables her to have lunch with her mother and be certain she is eating properly. It also gives her sufficient time to accompany Rita to the cemetery for a short visit.

12:15–1:00   Lunch with Jill.

1:00–1:45   Visit to cemetery.

1:45–2:30   Rita is to lie down and attempt to take a short nap. Normally she can't sleep, but she finds the time very relaxing and peaceful. She often reads during this passive rest period.

2:20–3:30   Housework and daily chores. Rita may leave the

home to get groceries, but generally doesn't want to drive anywhere alone.

3:30   Light carbohydrate recovery snack.

3:30–4:30   Scheduled visits with friends, talk on the telephone, or letter-writing.

4:30–5:30   Exercise by walking, doing light aerobics to a vid-
eotape made specifically for seniors, or attending a water aerobics
class. On Wednesday and Saturday, Jill accompanies Rita to a water
aerobics class for seniors. Rita has been taking water aerobics
classes for over a year but now refuses to go unless someone goes
with her. She finds the water exercise very satisfying and relaxing.
Exercising in the late afternoon has helped stabilize Rita's sleep cycle. She reports that she falls asleep easier and sleeps more deeply
when she exercises in the late afternoon.

5:30–6:00   Preparation of dinner with Jill.

6:00–7:30   Dinner and talk together. Jill reviews Rita's success at staying on the day's schedule and reviews the next day's
schedule in detail.

7:30   Jill returns home to spend the remainder of the evening
with her own family.

7:30–9:30   Reading, watching TV, talking on the phone, and
preparing meals and snacks for the next day.

9:30–10:00   Praying and reading the Bible.

10:00   Rita goes to bed. She has the numbers of several people to call should she need help or support during the night.

Summary, Rita

Rita must make the heartwrenching transition to widowhood from
a fulfilling marriage that she expected would continue for many
more years. Nothing can bring back the kind of happiness she lost,
but life offers other rewards to those who find the will and strength
to seize them.

The outlook for Rita's recovery is excellent. She has family,
friends, and strong religious beliefs and is free of financial worries.
In spite of all these advantages, however, without her daughter's determination to push Rita into vigorous recovery measures, Rita's recovery might be long delayed, or she might sink into chronic
depression.

Eric is 39, married with three children, ages 9, 12, and 15. He borrowed money from his father to start a small video production company. Eric previously worked as a technician for a local TV studio but had always dreamed of owning his own business.

His new company, however, is not doing well. He's out of capital and, after borrowing heavily from the bank, is nearly paralyzed by fear of failure and financial ruin. In addition, Eric feels unable to share his problems with his friends and family members. Even his wife doesn't know how severe their financial troubles are.

Eric reports that over the past few months he's been unable to relax, constantly worries, and is very irritable and negative. Recently, he reports feeling little or no energy, enthusiasm, or motivation. In Eric's own words, he's lost the desire and ability to "fight to stay above water."

Despite his lack of energy, he still works seven days a week—about 70 hours—at the studio "trying to get things right."

He spends very little time with his children, and when he does see them, he feels they are either antagonistic or indifferent to him. He regrets this, but frankly admits that he has neither the time nor the energy to "deal with it now." His wife is sympathetic, but concerned that her husband is "killing himself" with his work.

Although Eric has always been physically active and health-conscious, in the last three months his eating habits have deteriorated, and he has stopped exercising because he doesn't have time or energy for it. Eric says he is "less disciplined" about what and when he eats, and admits that cocktails at night are the only way he's been able to relax. Fifteen pounds overweight, Eric is disgusted and depressed by his "new body," but believes that he needs to put all his energy into his struggling business before he loses everything.

Toughness Training Interventions
Eric must balance the high volume of emotional stress associated with his failing business before he can perform at the high level of enthusiasm, energy, and competence it will take to turn his company around and put it on the road to success. To maximize Eric's

chances of accomplishing this, it is recommended that he adhere to the following schedule.

6:30 A.M.   Get up and dress for exercise.

6:30–7:00   Have a small glass of orange juice and prepare a "Things to Do" list for the day. Review previous day's unfinished items and establish a list of priorities. Most people report that creating such a list and ranking the items in order of importance significantly reduces their emotional stress. The reason for this is the increased sense of personal control and organization such lists provide.

7:00–7:30   Exercise for 30 minutes. Create as many cycles of stress and recovery as possible during the exercise by varying the intensity of jogging, walking, rebounding, or cycling. Go fast (stress), then slow (recovery), then fast again, etc. (See Chapter 9, "Getting Tough Physically".) Interval exercise provides Eric with numerous episodes of recovery to better understand and train his recovery mechanisms.

7:30–8:30   Shower, dress, and have breakfast (a carbohydrate-centered, low-fat, low-calorie meal). Eric is not allowed to skip breakfast as a strategy for losing weight.

8:30–10:30   Work. Eric is to adhere to his "Things to Do" list of priorities as much as possible.

10:30–10:45   Exercise and nutrition break. Eric's office is in a high-rise building. Using the building's internal stairway, he is to walk up four flights of stairs and down four flights for 10 minutes. Following the exercise, he is to consume half an apple or orange and drink four to six ounces of water.

10:45–12:30 P.M.   Work.

12:30–1:30   Lunch. Eric's lunch should be a low-fat, carbohydrate-dense meal containing no more than 500 calories. Examples would be pasta salad, fruit plate, or seafood salad.

1:30–3:00   Work.

3:00–3:20   Passive rest and nutrition break. Eric is to have his secretary hold all calls for 20 minutes. He closes the office door, removes a pad and blanket from his closet, and attempts to take a 15-minute nap. Relaxation is the goal; it doesn't matter whether he falls asleep or not. Eric sets a timer for 15 minutes, to allow him time to consume a no-fat carbohydrate snack following the rest period.

3:20–5:30   Work.

5:30–6:00   Have pure carbohydrate snack not to exceed 70 calories, review "Things to Do" list, make last-minute phone calls, and clean off desk before leaving.

6:00–7:00   Spend time with his kids doing some form of exercise. Examples would be kicking a soccer ball, throwing a Frisbee, or playing tennis. When playing and exercising with his children is not possible, Eric is to exercise on his own for a minimum of 20 minutes.

7:00–7:45   Dinner with his family. The goal for Eric is to eliminate all alcohol and to consume not more than 500 calories for this meal. Because Eric has been consuming some type of food about every two hours, he never gets overly hungry. It will be much easier for him to avoid overeating the way he has been doing in the past.

7:45–9:00   Eric is to spend time with his wife talking about the business and the day's activities. He also is to help his children with their homework when needed. Eric's goal is to become much more open with his wife regarding his fears and concerns about the business. Being able to talk about his feelings will provide emotional relief for Eric, reduce his feeling of aloneness, and strengthen his relationship with his wife.

9:00–10:00   Open, unstructured time. May watch TV, read the paper, make phone calls, work on household chores, and so on. When needed, this time can be used to talk further with his wife. Since the children are in bed by 9:00 P.M., this affords more privacy and freedom to talk openly.

10:00–10:30   Watch news and sports on TV.

10:30–6:30 A.M.   Sleep. Eric's goal is to sleep 8 hours each night. He is to record the number of hours of sleep and the quality of the sleep on a daily basis.

Summary, Eric

Eric's schedule is designed to accomplish several things. The first and most important is to stabilize his basic needs for physiological recovery. Carefully controlling the timing and content of his meals as well as the timing and the volume of his sleep provides this.

Eating some form of carbohydrate every two hours or so ensures better control of blood sugar levels. That means Eric will feel more sustained energy throughout the day, and because he never gets overly hungry, will be able to control his tendency to overeat. Eliminating alcohol and late-night meals also means fewer sleep problems and more complete sleep cycles.

The second most important objective regarding Eric's schedule is to provide relief from the excessive volume of emotional stress set off by his failing business. Eric's life-style has become increasingly linear: no exercise, constant work, no one to talk to, no time off, no fun. The signs of overtraining emotionally and undertraining physically are clearly evident. His fatigue, low motivation, poor concentration, inability to sleep, and constant feelings of pressure are classic symptoms.

Eric's ability to work effectively and efficiently, to think clearly, and to find real answers to his pressing financial problems has been seriously undermined by the excessive stress. His "Things to Do" list, scheduled exercise, afternoon naps, and improved communication with his wife and children form a stress-beating pattern. They all serve to reduce the overall volume of stress as well as induce waves of recovery that provide relief from his increasing linearity.

RAPED

Alice, 27 years old, is single and lives alone. She works as a teacher in a local elementary school and is completing her master's degree in elementary education at a nearby university. Awakened in the middle of the night by an intruder holding a knife to her throat, Alice was raped and beaten and had most of her personal jewelry stolen. She immediately reported the rape and theft to the police but found them to be very unresponsive, insensitive, and ineffectual.

One week after the rape, Alice reports feelings of extreme fear, anger, and depression. She indicates that she is constantly fearful of being raped again and has recurring nightmares of the rape incident.

Alice reports that she is afraid to go to bed at night, awakens frequently, and feels exhausted when morning finally arrives. She reports frequent crying sessions and extreme anger, and she strongly believes the rapist will return.

Just two weeks prior to the rape, Alice had broken up with a longtime boyfriend whom she had intended to marry. She ended the relationship when she discovered he had been sexually involved with another woman. Alice feels completely alone and isolated. She does not want her students or colleagues at work to know anything about the incident. She is very reluctant to talk about the rape with anyone except the police and a close personal friend.

Toughness Training Interventions

Alice's most pressing recovery need is for safety and security. The fear, which completely dominates her life at the current time, is potentially very destructive and is disruptive to most recovery mechanisms. In addition to stabilizing Alice's basic physiological needs for sleep and nutrition, fulfilling her needs for safety and security has the highest priority.

Based on her present situation, the following steps are recommended to minimize the destructive impact of the tragic life event.

1. STOP LIVING ALONE.

Alice should make immediate arrangements to stay with her longtime friend, who lives in the same city. She should not return to her apartment and live alone. Prior to the rape, Alice had been considering moving to a small house where she could keep a dog for companionship and protection. Now is the time to make that move. Alice needs as much relief as possible from her overpowering fear of being alone and getting raped again. Moving in with a friend, moving from the apartment where the rape occurred, and making plans for a guard dog provide immediate response to her needs for safety and security.

2. BEGIN THERAPY IMMEDIATELY.

Alice should carefully select a professional therapist who is experienced in working with rape victims. This is critical for her emotional recovery, because she has few people with whom she can openly discuss her strong feelings and emotions.

3. DON'T STOP WORKING.

Alice should continue teaching school if possible. Going to work, teaching, and working with children will force her to get her mind off the traumatic event. This actually works to give temporary relief from the stressor.

4. JOIN A SUPPORT GROUP.

If Alice can join or start a support group for victims of rape, she should do so. Between her group meetings, being able to openly talk about her anger, fear, and emotional pain with her friend daily will significantly speed up dissipation of the emotionally charged event and aid her in making a full recovery.

5. GET ENOUGH SLEEP.

The rape incident has seriously disrupted Alice's ability to get sufficient sleep. She awakens several times during the night and is often terrified by recurring nightmares. As a result she delays going to bed in the evening as long as possible even though she finds herself exhausted. Alice's lack of sleep is steadily undermining her capacity to adjust to the excessive volume of emotional stress. Reestablishing her nighttime sleep cycle is of great importance.

Here are recommended steps:

- Exercise vigorously for a full hour from 5:00 to 6:00 P.M. daily. Alice is to use a combination of exercise routines, including aerobic dance, walking, jogging, biking, tennis, and swimming to decrease nervous tension and experience emotional relief. Exercise in the early evening will help to stabilize Alice's sleep cycle.
- Get to bed early (10:00–10:30) and follow the same schedule daily.
- Avoid thinking or talking about emotionally charged issues after 9:00 P.M. Entertaining disruptive emotional thoughts and memories prior to going to bed can seriously interfere with falling asleep.
- Do whatever is possible to minimize the trauma of the nightmares. Leaving a light on in the bedroom, keeping a small TV on during the night, or allowing a pet to sleep in the same room can help reduce fear when suddenly awakened by a bad dream.
- Understand that nightmares are part of the healing process and will soon be over.

- Have a definite routine to follow when unable to get back to sleep—reading, meditating, praying, listening to music.
- Eat and drink nutritionally on a precise schedule. Avoid going more than 2½ hours without eating; choose light, low-fat, low-sugar snacks between carbohydrate-heavy meals. Finish with dinner no later than 7:30.

6. THE MOST DIFFICULT HEALING STEP: MAKE A DAILY SEARCH FOR POSITIVE MEANING.

As soon as Alice has organized her life to provide adequate safety, sleep, and nutrition, she should start working for a few minutes every day at trying to give some positive meaning to the tragic occurrence. She should ask herself each day, "What have I learned from it that can help me become a stronger, better, more resilient, more sensitive, and more responsive person?" This will never be easy—it will be very painful at first—but over time, if she works at it, the event can be a source of strength.

UNEMPLOYED

Peter, 48 years old, is married and has two children, ages 17 and 19. He has worked for the same manufacturing company for 16 years and for the last 4 years held a senior management position with the company.

Based on his longevity, his positive performance reviews, and his senior position, Peter expected to work at the company until he retired. However, along with nearly 5,000 other employees, Peter lost his job when the entire plant was closed. The news devastated him.

Peter has tried to find a comparable job for the last six months, with no success. With benefits, his income had been over $100,000 a year. Family savings are nearly gone, and Peter and his wife will have two children in college next year.

Peter's primary emotional responses to the crisis are anger and fear. He has lost most of his confidence and self-esteem because of the layoff and the consistent rejection he feels when attempting to market his skills. He is clearly losing hope for the future. His wife is sympathetic but increasingly less tolerant of Peter's negativism and failure to take positive action.

Peter's symptoms of excessive stress include mild to moderate depression, emotional withdrawal, irritability, weight gain, sleep problems, and periods of intense anxiety followed by low energy. He doesn't exercise, drinks four to eight ounces of alcohol every evening, and has cut himself off from most of his past friends because of his embarrassment at having no job.

Toughness Training Interventions

Peter's physical, emotional, and mental health are rapidly deteriorating. Immediate steps need to be taken to reverse his declining self-esteem, sense of helplessness, and fear of failure. With each passing month since the layoff, Peter's life has become increasingly linear. The traumatic event has clearly exceeded his coping skill and has led to progressive weakening. Peter's untrained response to the crisis and his poor recovery skills render him increasingly helpless. His defensiveness, low energy, persistent anger and fear, emotional detachment, and inability to act are clear markers of emotional overtraining.

Even though Peter tried hard to be positive and upbeat during employment interviews, his low self-esteem and weakened condition were clearly evident. Unless Peter can show more energy, enthusiasm, and strength in interviews, it is highly unlikely that he will be successful in the job market. More important, if Peter does not get relief from the extreme emotional stress and is unable to reverse the progressive weakening, he will likely suffer a complete mental and emotional breakdown.

Peter's weakened condition makes it unlikely that he will take the initiative to begin a comprehensive personal training program. His low motivation, fear of failure, and poor self-esteem will not allow it. The best way to get Peter to launch and adhere to a new training program is through his wife, Sandra. Although Peter's relationship with his wife increasingly is combative, he is deeply connected to her emotionally.

If Sandra indicates that she really needs his help to keep her head above water, Peter will probably respond. Her request would be for him to go on the Toughness Training program with her so that she will have the courage and strength to stay with it. Sandra needs to let Peter know that she can't make it alone. She desperately needs his help. The goal would be to launch a comprehensive program of mental, emotional, and physical toughening—*together.*

1. ESTABLISH A WELL-DEFINED, PRECISE DAILY SCHEDULE OF EATING AND SLEEPING.

2. ENTER A 30-DAY CRASH COURSE.
Set aside the next 30 days to toughen before attempting any new employment efforts. After the 30-day intensive training period, both Peter and Sandra will attempt to find employment.

3. BUY MORE TIME.
Take a second mortgage on the home to buy additional time and get relief from the financial pressure. Although nearly all their savings are gone, they have substantial equity in their home. If necessary, Peter and Sandra could sell their home and lease something smaller. This would substantially reduce financial pressures for some time even if both remain unemployed for several additional months.

4. WORK TO A DISCIPLINED SCHEDULE FOR 30 DAYS.
Establish an hour-by-hour schedule for the next 30 days that meets the following conditions:
- Set an optimal circadian sleep cycle. Up early and to bed early.
- Reduce alcohol consumption to no more than three ounces daily but none after 7:30 P.M. because of the impact alcohol has on Peter's sleep cycle. For the same reason, dinner should be light and finished by 8:00 P.M.

5. SHATTER LINEARITY.
Consciously work at breaking mental, emotional, and physical linearity. Make as many waves of stress and recovery as possible throughout the day. Attempt to create major stress and recovery waves every 90 to 120 minutes. If Peter has been watching TV for an hour and a half, he is to exercise, work in the garden, go shopping—anything that involves movement. If he has been experiencing great emotional stress, he is to break the cycle of stress by inducing an effective wave or recovery through some form of active or passive rest.

6. EXPAND ACTIVE AND PASSIVE REST OPTIONS.

During the next 30 days, Peter and Sandra are to add a minimum of three new active rest options and three new passive rest options that work for them. Explore golf, tennis, relaxation tapes, laugh tapes, video comedies, meditation, yoga, tai-chi, walking, swimming—the choices are many and varied. Enrolling in a yoga class is strongly recommended because it stimulates mental, emotional, and physical recovery.

Summary, Peter

The most serious consideration for Peter is that his cycle of excessive stress has lasted over six months with virtually no forward progress in any direction. A prolonged period of weakening and the accompanying linearity are deadly. Serious physical and mental health problems are likely if Peter's condition of excessive stress persists.

Because of his weakened state, Peter is incapable of initiating or sustaining any Toughness Training interventions by himself. Active involvement by Sandra is critical.

The first goal of the intervention process should be to reverse Peter's progressive weakening and linearity. This is initially done by faithfully fulfilling his basic physical recovery needs such as sleep, food, water, and movement. Once Peter's basic physical needs are stabilized, the training's focus should be shifted to structuring intermittent waves of emotional recovery with a wide variety of active and passive rest activities.

Talking, the therapy of renewing old friendships, and reducing financial pressures by obtaining a second mortgage will also help to increase the effectiveness and volume of recovery. Once the symptoms of excessive stress begin to disappear, Peter should use the information in Chapters 7, 9, and 10 to start a comprehensive program of mental, emotional, and physical toughening.

6

THE CHEMISTRY

OF TOUGHNESS—

SPIKING THE

RIGHT EMOTIONS

This chapter links Toughness Training with its foundations in what researchers have learned about the chemicals circulating in your blood.

If you want to skip this chapter because it's a bit technical, take it as an exercise in Mental Toughness Training and plow through it anyway.

Plunge in fearlessly. Keep in mind that you don't have to memorize any of the details—just give it your best read. Your review of this material will deepen your understanding of the toughening process and its connection to the physical body.

Definitions for many of the uncommon terms are given in the glossary at the back of the book. You may find it helpful to refer to them as you read.

While some areas discussed here remain controversial and theoretical, professional consensus exists for many of the biochemical components of the toughening model presented in this book.

The work of the University of Nebraska's Richard Dienstbier contributed greatly to this chapter. The first of his two most important scientific papers on the toughness model appeared in 1989 as "Arousal and Physiological Toughness: Implications for Mental and Physical Health" in the *Psychological Review.* The second appeared in 1991 in *Medicine and Science in Sports and Exercise* under the title "The Behavioral Correlates of Sympathoadrenal Reactivity: The Toughness Model."

The evolution of his physiological toughness model has been inspirational in my work and has led to many important insights. Although his model relies principally on correlational studies and is as yet largely theoretical, strong support for his toughening concepts can be found in a wide diversity of research.

KEY POINT:

TOUGHNESS IS AN ACQUIRED

BIOCHEMICAL ADAPTATION.

At the heart of Dienstbier's model is the contention that toughness, as opposed to helplessness, is essentially an acquired biochemical adaptation. Toughness, reflected in what he calls the challenge response, stems from a distinctive type of physiological arousal that is closely connected to the activation of specific positive emotions.

DIENSTBIER'S TWO TOUGHNESS INDICATORS

Dienstbier hypothesized that:

1. Low negative emotion in response to stress indicates toughness. Negative emotions include such feelings as fear, anger, anxiety, and sadness.

2. High positive emotion in response to stress also indicates toughness. Positive emotions include feeling up to a challenge or a fight, determination, and confidence.

According to Dienstbier, the pattern of learned physiological arousal and its accompanying emotional state becomes the determining factor in toughness. One specific pattern of arousal in response to stress is called SNS-adrenal-medullary arousal.

This pattern starts with the release of two powerful hormones called epinephrine (EPI) and norepinephrine (NE). These two are part of the family of chemicals called catecholamines.

CATECHOLAMINES IN YOUR BLOOD

The catecholamines epinephrine and norepinephrine are often called adrenaline and noradrenaline. They are produced by the adrenal glands, which are found on top of the kidneys. Catecholamines are released by one of the adrenal system's two components, the adrenal medulla. The catecholamines have a powerful effect on metabolic rate, muscle activity, and the cardiovascular and nervous systems.

The release of the catecholamines occurs in response to mental stress, emotional stress, and physical exercise. As an example, working on a challenging math problem can cause a catecholamine release that dramatically increases blood flow, oxygen to the brain, and glucose supply. Muscle activity is also enhanced as a result of these changes.

Epinephrine (EPI) increases heart and metabolic rates and also causes glucose release.

Norepinephrine (NE) constricts the body's blood vessels and increases blood pressure. Along with the release of the adrenal steroid hormones called glucocorticoids, norepinephrine release during muscle activity helps the body convert fat to energy more easily.

TWO FUNDAMENTAL RESPONSES: CHALLENGE AND FEAR

The adrenal cortex produces over 30 steroid hormones called corticosteroids. The precise effect of all these hormones has not yet been conclusively established; however, much knowledge about them has already been acquired.

For example, while other hormones, such as the glucocorticoids, are important as well, the adrenal-medullary pattern is associated with increased energy and positive emotion. This is broadly described as *the challenge response.*

An entirely different pattern is associated with increased negative emotion—most often fear and tension. Cortisol is one of the two major corticosteroids produced by the adrenal cortex and is generally released when situations are perceived as threatening. This is called the pituitary-adrenal-cortical arousal, commonly recognized as *the fear response.*

CATECHOLAMINES, TOUGHNESS, AND PEAK PERFORMANCE

A number of Scandinavian researchers have reported a connection between catecholamine increases (EPI and NE) and improved performance on a wide variety of tasks. As an example, Swedish children who performed best on a math test showed hormonal increases in NE rather than decreases. Children with NE decreases clearly made more mistakes and had less work endurance.

A Finnish study found that NE increases correlate strongly with exam performance by high school students. Students with the largest increases in catecholamine activity did best on the exam. Similar results have been obtained with college students as well as with adults.

One of the most interesting and extensive studies was conducted with Norwegian army paratroopers. Catecholamine tests were made just before and after jumping from a training tower. Testing was also done before and after jumping from aircraft. Better performance was strongly associated with increases in EPI and NE. Poor performance was linked to the presence of blood cortisol, suggesting a different kind of physiological arousal from that experienced by the paratroopers who performed best.

Similar findings regarding catecholamines and cortisol were found in studies conducted during basic training of U.S. Navy recruits. Both American and Scandinavian studies have found that responsiveness in terms of catecholamine reactivity is associated with emotional stability. (Reactivity is the ability to increase catecholamine levels quickly and sensitively in response to stress.) This finding is particularly important in the context of emotional responsiveness discussed in Chapter 1.

THE BASIS OF EMOTIONAL RESILIENCY

Catecholamine responsivity appears to be critical to effective coping. Of great interest also was the finding that emotional stability, superior performance, and low anxiety are associated with rapid declines in catecholamine levels. This confirms the importance of fast hormonal recovery.

In Toughness Training, rapid catecholamine decline may well be the physiological basis for emotional resiliency. Some research findings also suggest a connection between emotional strength and catecholamine response.

Both emotional stability and superior performance have been associated with two measurable—and closely linked—factors:

1. Low levels of catecholamines during rest periods
2. High levels of catecholamines once the stressor situation is introduced

Chronically high catecholamine levels (often associated with chronic feelings of stress) prevent a dramatic rise in these hormones. A strong, positive emotional response to challenging stressors may well be linked to one's ability to spike catecholamine levels from low to high.

Again, this supports the importance of biochemical recovery. Without low resting levels, spiking the chemistry to produce a strong challenge response may not be possible.

THE TOUGHENING PROCESS

In the early 1960s, several researchers explored the effects of environmental stimulation and stress on young animals. Rats and mice were regularly exposed to different schedules of such things as handling, mother separation, and electroshock. A surprising finding was that the animals exposed to daily stressors had larger adrenal glands as adults, but were less fearful and frightened when exposed to threats than the protected control group.

These studies were the first to link stressor stimulation during childhood with later adult emotional stability and stress tolerance. In 1976, W. D. Pfeifer discovered that although stimulated animals had larger and heavier adrenal glands, they surprisingly had lower resting levels of both catecholamine and cortisol.

Even more significant was the finding that during stressful situations, animals receiving early stimulation tended to be calmer, produced lower cortisol levels, and were able to spike catecholamines from low resting rates to high. They were also able to return quickly to resting rates.

About the same time that Pfeifer conducted his research on catecholamine and cortisol responses, J. M. Weiss discovered that low levels of a brain catecholamine, norepinephrine, is associated with animal helplessness. When drugs were administered that would block norepinephrine depletion, helplessness ceased. Depletion of this brain catecholamine seemed clearly linked to helplessness and what might be termed nontough behavior. Weiss concluded that chronic stress that permitted little or no recovery time was the primary cause of the catecholamine depletion.

The next logical step for Weiss was to determine the effect of intermittent exposure to stress in which numerous opportunities for recovery existed. He suspected that cycles of intermittent stress that provided ample time for recovery might actually increase tolerance for stress and resistance to norepinephrine depletion.

Weiss and his associates tested this assumption by exposing animals to intermittent cold-water swimming and uncontrollable electric shock over a period of fourteen days. After the fourteenth day of training the animals were subjected to the same potent stressors that they were exposed to at the onset of the study.

As predicted, no drop in performance or evidence of helplessness was observed. The results clearly showed that the animals had "toughened up" as a result of the intermittent training stress. Examination of the brains of the trained animals verified that the intermittent waves of stress prevented catecholamine depletion, confirming the critical role of recovery in the toughening process.

Researchers also discovered that animal "toughening" could be accomplished by exposing the animals to any number of passive and active stressors. Passive stressors such as electric shock, exposure to cold, loud noises, and regular handling—as well as active stressors such as aerobic exercise—all resulted in increased stress tolerance.

Any of those stressors, however, could lead to decreased stress tolerance and nontough behavior when the animals were stressed too severely or when insufficient time for recovery was provided.

Overcrowding is an example of a passive stressor that did not result in toughening because the animals were unable to achieve relief from the stress. Because the effect of crowding was constant, adequate recovery could not be achieved.

TAKING THE PAIN OUT OF FEAR'S BITE: CONTROLLING CORTISOL

To become challenged is to become positively aroused. Positive arousal in response to stress represents the core of toughness. Increased positive feelings of being ready for a fight, having energy, determination, aggressiveness, and so on correspond to increases in catecholamine levels.

To become threatened is to become negatively aroused. The feelings associated with negative arousal are linked to a variety of nontough response patterns. Researchers have identified the stress hormone cortisol as being strongly correlated with negative arousal. Both animal and human studies have confirmed the connection.

High levels of cortisol point to excessive stress. Sudden increases generally reflect the perception of threat and are associated with feelings of anxiety and fear. Chronically high levels of cortisol have been associated with depression, defensiveness, helplessness, neurosis, and even anorexia.

The control of cortisol appears to be related to past toughening experiences and one's perceived chances for successful coping in a particular situation. The perception that coping limits have been exceeded or that effective coping options are no longer available generally leads to immediate increases in cortisol levels.

High cortisol levels are typically experienced as very unpleasant and uncomfortable. However, when catecholamine increases without an increase in cortisol, no discomfort is experienced.

KEY POINT:

CATECHOLAMINE SPIKES LEAD TO EFFORT WITHOUT DISTRESS.

CORTISOL SPIKES LEAD TO EFFORT WITH DISTRESS.

One last significant research finding regarding cortisol was the fact that physically fit individuals are distinguished from unfit individuals by their ability to:

- Reduce cortisol levels more rapidly after it has been released
- Sustain positive challenge arousal for longer periods of time
- Delay large cortisol responses longer

The control of cortisol and other hormonal messengers associated with negative arousal plays a major role in the toughening process. Energy without distress keeps us moving forward until answers and solutions to the crisis can be found. Cortisol control is critical to both emotional control and the control of one's Ideal Performance State.

HOW CORTISOL CONTROL IS ACHIEVED

Cortisol control springs from mental and physical toughness, qualities that can be built by:

- Developing positive thinking skills, humor skills, tough beliefs, tough values, and similar mental attributes
- Increasing physical toughness in the form of physical fitness, plus learning to act and look tough under pressure

SUMMARY

Mental, emotional, and physical toughness are closely linked to learned patterns of arousal. To be tough is to respond physiologically to life events in a highly specific way.

Tough individuals are consistently able to perceive stressful situations as opportunities for growth, an attitude leading to what might best be referred to as the challenge response. The perception of challenge leads to a complex chain of biochemical events that mobilize the body to cope successfully with the stressor.

The physiological mobilization process associated with the perception of challenge is called *positive arousal*. Individuals lacking toughness are prone to perceive difficult life events as threatening and potentially harmful. The perception of threat leads to a condition of *negative arousal*, which is experienced as unpleasant and unenjoyable.

Evidence exists linking negative arousal with the stress hormone cortisol, which is produced by the adrenal cortex. Cortisol has been associated with feelings of anxiety, tension, helplessness, depression, and loss of control. Positive arousal, which is typically experienced as pleasant and enjoyable, has been linked to two powerful hormones produced by the adrenal medulla called epinephrine and norepinephrine. These hormones, referred to as the catecholamines, appear to be the principal physiological activators of the challenge response so typical of toughened individuals.

Toughness is related to several developed biochemical capacities, including the ability to:

- Produce an ample supply of the catecholamines
- Suppress cortisol release
- Maintain low catecholamine levels during normal, nonstressful times
- Powerfully spike catecholamine levels during coping periods
- Remain sensitive and responsive in one's tissue cells to catecholamine stimulation
- Rapidly reduce catecholamine levels following removal of the stressor

These catecholamine considerations provide a biochemical basis for the indicators of emotional toughness introduced in Chapter 1 (emotional flexibility, responsiveness, strength, and resiliency). The capacity for positive arousal, so typical of the toughened person, is clearly influenced by environmental factors.

From all the available research, the ideal toughening process is intermittent exposure to periods of stress followed by well-defined, regular periods of recovery. Repeated exposure to stress is necessary to increase catecholamine capacity (remember that stimulation causes adrenal glands to increase in size and weight), and it appears critical in the development of catecholamine sensitivity and responsiveness.

Sufficient recovery time is necessary to prevent catecholamine depletion as well as to strengthen catecholamine recovery mechanisms (return to low resting levels). When effective recovery follows cycles of stress, the perception of threat is not reinforced.

Recovery sends a vital message: "I'm OK." That message paves the way for the perception of challenge and positive arousal in similar future situations. Stress that leads to toughening can be either active or passive.

Active toughening results from deliberately seeking and structuring cycles of stress specifically for the purpose of accelerating the toughening process. Examples of such activities that have been linked to increased catecholamine production include physical exercise, competitive sport, and any number of emotional challenges.

Passive toughening results from using normal life stress to accelerate the toughening process. Challenging life events can clearly be used to toughen catecholamine response capabilities and enhance future coping skills. Of particular importance is the understanding that protection from stress diminishes catecholamine capacity, responsiveness, and sensitivity. Excessive, chronic stress leads to catecholamine depletion and recovery failure.

Too little or too much stress prevents the biochemical adaptations necessary for toughening. Producing toughness means exposure to cycles of balanced stress and recovery over time. Toughened individuals seem to thrive on stress. Rather than avoiding stress, they deliberately seek it out, and because of their acquired arousal control skills, they are able to stay positive, perform well, and remain challenged throughout a wide range of stressful circumstances.

They have learned to spike their chemistry when appropriate and necessary in stressful situations, resulting in powerful feelings of having energy, positive readiness to fight, and intensity. This mobilization process is the basis for successful coping and problem-solving.

7

GETTING TOUGH

EMOTIONALLY

Emotionally tough does not mean emotionally hard, cold, insensitive, or calloused. It simply means being in control, as opposed to being controlled.

Being tough emotionally means being able to deal with life in flexible, responsive, strong, and resilient ways. It means you control your emotions rather than the other way around. It means you can weather life's storms and seize life's opportunities. It means that when the going gets tough, you're tougher.

THE BASIC PREMISE OF EMOTIONAL TOUGHENING

Emotional toughening begins with a basic premise: The most natural, normal state of humankind is positive.

This is to say that a positive emotional state should be the norm rather than the exception. Man is designed to function best when his psychological and physiological needs can be registered against a positive state of mind.

A persistent and enduring positive emotional state is generally a reflection of balance and health. Emotions are mind/body talk. Just as positive emotions reflect balance, negative emotions reflect imbalance. When stress/recovery needs are adequately met, positive emotional states typically prevail.

However, positive emotional states must not be blindly pursued. It's critical to understand that all negative emotions serve a purpose—each and every one signals an unmet need of some kind.

Getting tougher emotionally can be accelerated in two ways: by getting tougher physically, as we will see in Chapter 9, and by getting tougher mentally, as we will see in Chapter 10. However, the present chapter focuses on the essential business of deciphering the messages being sent via the chemical messengers that negative emotions trigger.

The chemical messengers have something to say, and before you block the message, listen for the reason or purpose behind it.

When negative arousal occurs, here are the questions you should ask yourself:

1. WHAT IS THE RECOVERY NEED BEING EXPRESSED?
Exactly why am I angry, upset, depressed, frustrated, tired, and feeling negative?

2. CAN I DO ANYTHING ABOUT IT NOW?
If you can, attempt to meet the need as directly and constructively as possible. If you can't meet the need now, do you want to continue to feel this way? Is feeling angry or depressed meeting some additional emotional need—such as punishing a spouse or getting even with a coworker?

3. IS THIS THE RIGHT TIME AND PLACE FOR ME TO BE EXPERIENCING ALL THIS NEGATIVE EMOTION (PAIN)?
If it's occurring at work or during a competitive event such as a golf game or a tennis match, it's clearly *not* the right time. Negative emotional states during performances generally serve only to undermine the performance.

If this is not the right time or place, make a conscious, deliberate decision to change your emotional state. The strategies presented in this book will equip you with the tools to make that happen. But first, listen to and interpret the message.

For example, ask yourself, "Are the negative feelings I am now having the consequence of essentially irrational, nontough thinking?" Such thoughts as:

"I should always win."

"Everyone should like me."

"Nobody likes me."

If that's the case, take responsibility for the feelings and begin immediately to use your toughness tools to change from a negative to a positive state of mind.

4. IS THE PAIN THE RESULT OF TOUGH TIMES—FINANCIAL CRISIS, ILLNESS, OR A SIMILAR TRAUMA?

If so, ask yourself: Are my negative emotions helping? Can I use these stressful times to toughen emotionally? Can I become challenged by this crisis and get stronger rather than weaker because of this stress? If there's any way you can, make the decision to do exactly that.

5. ARE THE NEGATIVE FEELINGS SIGNALING GENUINE, UNMET RECOVERY NEEDS?

What are they? For sleep, food, love, attention, and such things? If so, make every effort to meet those needs as directly, constructively, and quickly as possible.

EMOTIONS ARE MIND/BODY TALK

Emotional toughening means gaining control over cycles of negative arousal (pituitary adrenal-cortical stimulation). To do that we have to tune in to the talk that goes on between mind and body. Let's take a closer look at how that's done.

The channels run both ways: mind to body, body to mind. The amazingly complex subtlety of these swift, vital, and multiple lines of continuous communication still poses vast mysteries that researchers are only slowly penetrating. But already we know a great deal that's important to Toughness Training.

POSITIVE EMOTIONS

Positive emotions indicate that the mind and body are in harmony. Everyone's normal state of mind should be positive—we were meant to be happy, confident, and energetic most of the time. However, these conditions are not likely to occur unless both stress and recovery needs are being adequately met.

NEGATIVE EMOTIONS

Negative emotions—pain, fear, guilt, anger, frustration, mental fatigue, hunger, thirst—indicate imbalance. These and the many other negative emotions signal that recovery needs are not being met. The more intense the negative emotion—as, for example, when it passes beyond discomfort into pain—the greater the need for recovery.

EMOTIONAL CONTROL

Becoming sensitive to our feelings is the first step toward commanding them instead of acting blindly on their impulses. We want to use emotions to our advantage instead of allowing them to push us into bad choices that will harm or defeat us. Emotions are the key to productivity, health, and happiness. Therefore, to control our lives we must learn to control our emotions.

LISTEN AND ANALYZE

First we must learn to listen and analyze the messages our emotions send us. It seems that few people think of listening to their emotions, of analyzing the messages, of consciously discarding the unhelpful and using only the helpful ones. We all do that to some degree (otherwise we would soon be behind bars), but few of us do it consciously according to a well-thought-out plan.

Unfortunately, many plans to control emotion rely on blocking out feelings. This serious mistake causes us to lose track of our needs. We have to do better than that to make emotional control the powerful toughening force it can be.

Without feelings and emotions we have no way to manage the

stress/recovery relationship. Need fulfillment makes that relationship work.

MESSENGERS, NOT CONTROLLERS

Keep in mind that feelings and emotions should be messengers, not controllers. They are the body's internal eyes and ears, the instrument gauges of the stress/recovery balance that is required not only for growth but even for survival. Think of feelings and emotions as flight data from Mission Control, faithfully guiding your journey through life. They will do that if you control them instead of being controlled by them.

The chatter (instrument data from your personal Mission Control) comes in continuously. It's always going: I feel tired, hungry, happy, bored, excited, depressed, threatened, scared, challenged, and a thousand other things.

TRANSLATION TIME

Many people instantly translate most of the messages sent by feelings and emotions into words; others simply feel them. Some of us need to enhance our ability to distinguish between situations calling for either response.

When physical action is involved, there's usually no time for the translation into words—we respond instantly or it's too late. In other situations, especially when the indicated response will be in spoken words, we have enough time for the translation.

We all occasionally see hot-tempered people fail to consider the consequences of their words before speaking them. It's a common cause of disaster in everyday life, and also in sport. Athletes are trained for instant reaction to make a double play or return serve. When they respond the same way to what they consider an umpire's or linesman's bad call, they often knock themselves out of their Ideal Performance State.

NEGATIVE FEELINGS INDICATE IMBALANCE

If the emotion is a negative feeling—either a physical or a psychological one—it indicates imbalance. The imbalance could be too little stress against too much recovery, but more often it reflects too much stress against insufficient recovery.

Mild negative emotion (slight discomfort) indicates a mild recovery need. Severe negative emotion (pain) indicates a serious recovery need.

HOW HEALTHY PEOPLE REACT TO NEGATIVE EMOTIONS

Healthy people know what they want. They're decisive. That means that they understand their feelings very well.

It's a lot harder than it sounds.

Feelings can be very confusing. Often they are puzzling, coming as they do from many directions. Deciphering the legitimate needs that lie behind these sometimes bizarre feelings can be difficult.

Toughness is shown by people who know what they want, know their feelings, are decisive, and are able to respond correctly.

A healthy person consistently sees through and ignores unimportant feelings while at the same time correctly interpreting and responding to genuine and appropriate needs.

Being able to read one's feelings and understand what are the needs behind those feelings is an important life skill. It's a skill that enables a person to distinguish between trivial or unwholesome need feelings that should be ignored, and legitimate needs that must be met. These feelings often take a variety of strange forms— sometimes it takes patient detective work to pin down what the source of the imbalance is.

The skill lies in separating essential from nonessential needs and fulfilling the legitimate needs directly and constructively.

THE CRITICAL RULE OF PERSONAL AWARENESS

A prerequisite of emotional health and need fulfillment is a highly developed sense of personal awareness. Healthy, toughened people are acutely aware of the messages their minds and bodies are sending via feelings, sensations, and emotions. A good analogy is Mission Control Center at Cape Canaveral during a shuttle space mission. A wide variety of critical flight factors are constantly and carefully monitored at all times. An alert, highly focused flight controller tracking an array of sophisticated computer monitors is analogous to the toughened person tracking stress and recovery with a keen sense of personal awareness.

The computer screens of healthy people are relatively clear, indicating things are generally balanced and positive. Unmet needs, which represent stress, appear on the computer screen in the form of negative feelings and sensations that are in varying degrees unpleasant. Negative thinking and feelings, ranging from mild discomfort to intense pain, signal unmet needs of various kinds and call for IMMEDIATE ATTENTION and possible IMMEDIATE ACTION.

When important needs remain unmet, the cycle of stress is perpetuated, thus increasing the risks of overtraining and sustained negativism. Chronic negativism blunts awareness. Systems become overloaded; distress signals become impossible to trace; alarms become empty messages. Chronic negativism is the consequence of repeated failure to meet important needs and virtually guarantees that needs will remain unmet.

In the healthy, toughened person, the sequence goes like this: A positive mental state is momentarily interrupted when negative, unpleasant feelings break into awareness. Attention is then immediately directed to the source of the discomfort. What is the need being expressed? Is it important or unimportant? Can the need be fulfilled now or later? If the need is judged to be important, a commitment is made to fulfill the need as quickly and constructively as possible. Fulfillment of the need brings relief and balance.

Toughened people are those who are sensitive to their needs, have learned to understand and recognize them for what they are, and can fulfill those needs in direct, healthy ways. Developing a keen sense of personal awareness is indispensable to that process.

HOW UNHEALTHY PEOPLE REACT TO NEGATIVE EMOTIONS

In contrast to the healthy person, who has a decisive and positive reaction to a negative emotion and meets it head-on, unhealthy people react with utter confusion. Typically they respond in ways that do not even remotely begin to meet the need behind the negative feeling. Often the confused response is repeated each time the negative emotion is felt, each time leaving the person worse off than before.

For example, self-esteem needs often get confused. The confusion can become very complex. Anorexic women feel their self-esteem needs so profoundly that they block out their body's craving for adequate nourishment and literally starve themselves to death. The many cases of anorexia nervosa provide well-publicized proof that misinterpreting a negative emotion can be lethal. Similarly, needs for love and affection, especially when they are strong, sometimes cause confused responses, such as sexual promiscuity or overeating.

Suppose we are depressed. The depression signals a need. We must identify the real need and meet it rather than mask it by doing something that may give momentary relief (such as overeating) or merely shuts off the message (such as abusing alcohol or using drugs). Since none of these measures meets the real need, they are bound to fail, thus leaving us worse off than before.

There are other signals of unmet needs. Being overly aggressive often signals a need. For example, during a phone conversation a salesman says something that really irritates you. Somewhat to your surprise, you really rip into the guy. What this can really mean is that you're touchy because you're under too much stress and need some recovery time.

Chewing the other guy out might give you momentary relief, but it does no lasting good and may be harmful by making you feel guilty. What you should do is listen to the message that your negative emotion is trying to send you, and get in some good recovery time. Go home and play with your kids; take the wife to dinner. Go fishing. Take a swim, or jog, or take a few days of vacation time.

HOW NEGATIVE AROUSAL CAN HELP YOU

In some situations you can't get into your Ideal Performance State without first going through a period of negative arousal. Gifted stage performers often go through a painful period of nervousness before appearing in front of an audience. Many highly successful artists consider this to be a necessary step that psyches them up to give a superior performance.

Some performers destroy their careers by masking the psychological pain of preperformance jitters with drugs or alcohol. Others experiment with mental relaxation techniques that either leave them emotionally flat and uninspired when they step out on stage or intensify their nervousness during their performances.

It seems that nervousness before a performance often translates into calm control during the performance. This appears to be true in cases of stage performances and public speaking; it may be particularly important in sport competition.

Someone who pretends that the competition or the performance will be no big deal—never thinks about it beforehand, merely relaxes ahead of time—may experience a strong anxiety response during the competition or performance.

In other words, moderate preperformance anxiety correlates with positive performance when it counts.

Recent research strongly supports this view. Anne Manyande and others at St. Marks Hospital in London studied surgery patients and relaxation training aimed at decreasing preoperative and postoperative distress. One group of patients received presurgery relaxation training; a control group did not. Manyande writes of her study that "the results suggest that preoperative relaxation increased the stressfulness of surgery."

Manyande's surprising conclusion shows that negative emotions often have vital roles to play. It means that we should channel our anxieties toward psyche-up rather than attempt to mask or deny them.

EMPOWERING VS. DISEMPOWERING EMOTIONS

To achieve maximum productivity, health, and happiness, develop your ability to access empowering emotions at will. Also learn to block out and ignore—that is, control—disempowering emotions.

However, we must learn to distinguish between disempowering emotions that indicate long-term stress/recovery imbalance and negative feelings that report immediate unfulfilled bodily needs. During performances—both in life and in sport—you can't repair long-term stress/recovery imbalance. Your opportunities to answer unfulfilled bodily needs may also be limited.

In many cases, however, hearing the message and realizing its importance can inspire you to meet those bodily needs. They range between easily met things, such as standing up and stretching if you've been sitting at a desk for a long time, and things you frequently can't meet immediately, such as needing sleep. If you can't fill the need right away, tell yourself that you will as soon as possible, and concentrate on the opportunity at hand.

EMPOWERING EMOTIONS

Empowering emotions generally indicate stress/recovery balance and health. Among these are:

Excitement	Passion	Determination
Spirit	Energy	Confidence
Challenge	Motivation	Drive
Resolution	Happiness	Enthusiasm

DISEMPOWERING EMOTIONS

Disempowering emotions generally indicate long-term stress/recovery imbalance—that is, unfilled needs for recovery. Among these are:

Fear	Anger	Helplessness
Guilt	Fatigue	Loneliness
Insecurity	Confusion	Exhaustion
Inadequacy	Depression	Ineptitude

NEGATIVE FEELINGS

Negative feelings generally indicate short-term stress/recovery imbalance—usually unfilled bodily needs. Among these are:

Hunger	Thirst	Fatigue
Discouragement	Lack of energy	Weakness

RECOVERY EMOTIONS

Recovery emotions generally indicate that recovery is taking place. Among these are:

Relaxation	Calmness	Rest
Tranquillity	Peace	Quiet

EMOTIONAL CONTROL

The key fact to remember is that we can control our emotional state at any given time—we don't have to be at the mercy of our feelings and emotions. To gain control, take the following steps:

1. Listen to the negative feelings.
2. Take the message.
3. Translate the message—that is, determine what recovery needs are not being met.
4. Commit to meeting the unfulfilled needs as quickly and constructively as possible.
5. Return to a positive emotional state, and for problem-solving or maximum performance, return to an empowered emotional state.
6. Seize control with positive thoughts.

For example, suppose you have just finished a long trip and are suffering from jet lag. To gain control you might go through the steps this way:

1. Sense the emotion: "I'm feeling tired and irritable."
2. Grasp the information: "OK, I'll take the message."
3. Analyze the message: "What needs are not being met? Let's see, I got only three hours' sleep last night because of the late flight, and I haven't eaten anything for over three hours. That means my blood sugar is probably low."
4. Commit to later action to meet a bodily need: "I'll go to bed early tonight, and sleep at least nine hours."
5. Take immediate action to meet a bodily need: "I'm going to break for lunch right now."

6. Seize control with positive thoughts: "I got the message. I'm tired and hungry, and I'll take care of both items as soon as I can—but for right now I choose to return to a positive emotional state."

THE PHONE IS RINGING

Negative emotions are like a phone ringing in your body. Don't block the call; instead, give it a clear line into your brain.

When negative emotions start surfacing and your internal-feelings phone is ringing—pick it up. A ringing phone indicates a need for recovery. Minor needs are signaled by soft rings—that is, by light negative emotions or feelings. You feel mildly irritated, hungry, tired, bored, or something similar. Urgent needs are signaled by loud, painful rings—by strong negative emotions such as intense fear, anger, depression, hopelessness, exhaustion, or something else with similar impact.

The feelings and emotions you're hearing are stress/recovery talk. Work at learning the skill of understanding and interpreting the meanings of negative emotions. A ringing phone—your awareness of negative emotion—serves a critical role. If you don't get the message and respond in ways that fulfill the need, the phone will continue to ring. It will get louder and louder (cause you more and more pain) as time goes on without the need being met.

GUARANTEEING TROUBLE

Denying that your internal-feelings phone is ringing, or blocking out the pain with alcohol or other drugs, is like refusing to answer the phone at work or home. This action guarantees that your recovery needs won't be met.

A fundamental fact is that failing to meet one's critical recovery needs will eventually have dire consequences. One of the most dramatic examples of this is the feeling of helplessness and low self-esteem that sometimes drives people to suicide.

Short of such tragedies, the price of disconnecting can still be disastrously high in terms of unhappiness, lost health, and low productivity. Listening to the body through feelings and emotions is essential for self-management and self-regulation.

OVERDOING A GOOD THING

However, listening to the body's feelings and emotions can easily be overdone. Some people become chronically negative, meaning that nearly all the time negative emotions are flowing through their brains wreaking destruction. This means their phones are constantly ringing with unmet needs.

In some cases the chronically negative condition stems from consistently failing to satisfy bodily needs—as the undernourished alcoholic does because liquor masks his hunger for food. In other cases it arises because the person dwells constantly on negative thoughts not necessarily related to unmet bodily needs.

For both kinds of chronically negative people, negative is normal rather than the reverse. Extreme cases can no longer decipher their recovery needs because their phone is always ringing, and the messages are completely lost in all the background noise. Their needs simply don't get met, and imbalance becomes the norm.

Chronic negativism results from habitually ignoring the ringing phone, from not taking the message, and from failing to do anything about it. This means the individual's needs can't be met, so he or she is always in pain.

We must hear the ring before it becomes too obnoxiously urgent, because if we wait that long, weakening will already have taken place. Always take the message, and respond to the need as soon as possible.

ANSWERING THE PHONE AND GETTING OFF THE HOOK

Once we answer the phone—once we tune in to the negative emotions and take the message—there's no need for the phone to keep on ringing (that is, there's no reason for us to remain in a negative emotional state). As of that instant, we're free to put ourselves back in a positive emotional state that will help us achieve our objective of the moment.

To get off the hook we must:

1. Hear the phone announcing the negative feeling
2. Take the message reporting physical or psychological pain (par-

ticularly in cases of psychological pain, it's best to write the cause down)

3. Fulfill the need, or the phone will start ringing again, only this time it will ring louder, reflecting more pain.

Remember, this is essentially the only way your body has of getting your attention and making you take the necessary steps to supply its physical and psychological needs.

MAKING BEING POSITIVE YOUR NORMAL STATE

Being totally positive all the time is not normal. It's not healthy, because it means that somehow you are preventing the phone from ringing. As a result you never get all your body's essential messages.

The golden rule is: *Become sensitive to your body.* When it calls, pick up the phone and respond accordingly. Doing this means that being positive will become your normal state. You will listen to your negative emotions, get the message, and return immediately to your positive state.

To make this work you must do your best to meet the needs as directly and quickly as possible. If you don't pay attention to the ringing phone and things continue to worsen, you may get an abusive or obscene phone call from your body, or even a death threat. That's if you're lucky. If you're unlucky, something will mask the abusive call or death threat. You won't get the message, and the threatened injury or illness will strike.

FIVE STEPS FOR TAKING EMOTIONAL CONTROL

Here is my five-step formula for taking emotional control of your life:

STEP 1
When the phone starts ringing (when you start feeling negative), answer the phone by asking, "What am I feeling?" For example, are you sad, lonely, depressed, tired, angry, or what?

STEP 2

What is the unfulfilled need? Is it physical, mental, or emotional? Write it down. Be as specific as possible. If you're not sure, take a guess.

STEP 3

Tell yourself, "Thanks for the call," and commit to yourself that you will fulfill the need as soon as possible in the healthiest and most appropriate way.

STEP 4

Change your emotional state back to a positive one—an empowering one, if possible. You received the message your body was sending—you answered the phone, so it doesn't need to keep ringing. Now there's no need to feel negative anymore—you've done all that can be done at the moment.

KEY POINT:

YOU HAVE A MUCH BETTER CHANCE OF FINDING HEALTHY WAYS TO

FULFILL YOUR NEEDS WHEN YOU FEEL POSITIVE AND EMPOWERED.

IF YOU'RE NOT, USE YOUR MENTAL AND PHYSICAL TOUGHNESS SKILLS

TO CHANGE YOUR CHEMISTRY AND GET BACK TO FEELING POSITIVE.

HERE ARE SOME OF THE THINGS YOU CAN DO: CHANGE YOUR

THINKING, USE HUMOR, EXERCISE, STRETCH, ACT "AS IF."

STEP 5

After you change your emotional state to a positive state— preferably an empowered one—begin to problem-solve how best to meet your most pressing unfulfilled recovery needs. Then put your best plan *into action*.

──────────── **TAKE THE MESSAGE, MOVE ON** ────────────

That's how you get emotional control—not by blocking negative feelings, not by denying them, not by covering them up. You simply receive the intended message and return to your normal, positive state. When you do that, there's no reason to make everyone around you miserable with your phone ringing off the wall. The message your body is sending has nothing to do with making a scene of your negativeness. Take the message and move on!

THE EMOTIONS ASSOCIATED WITH STRESS AND RECOVERY

Figure 7.1 represents four stages of stress and two of recovery in one complete stress/recovery cycle.

1. *Undertraining.* Subject is conscious of mild stress, feels a little slow, maybe a little lazy, has low energy. Feels need for energy expenditure or stress, but very low need for recovery.
2. *Maintenance stress.* Normal energy expenditure, reaching the

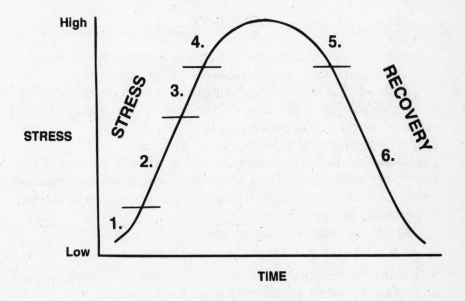

Figure 7.1   How You Feel During Various Levels of Stress and Recovery

Ideal Performance State, is easiest here. Subject has positive feelings that are easy to balance. Slight need for recovery.

3. *Toughening stress.* Subject feels challenged, uncomfortable, pushed, and is aware of mild physical or psychological pain that is adaptive. Strong recovery needs.

4. *Overtraining.* Marked by excessive stress that causes real pain. Subject has an immediate, intense need for recovery. The pain can be either physical or psychological—for example, it can include exhaustion, depression, fear, anger, and feelings of helplessness.

5. *Partial recovery.* Subject experiences a tremendous feeling of relief at this stage, but recovery mechanisms such as sleep often fail under conditions of high stress.

6. *Full recovery.* recovery needs are being met. Subject feels calm, relaxed, relieved, rested, and fulfilled, either physically or emotionally.

SUMMARY

Excessive stress produces pain. Negative emotion is the vehicle through which pain is communicated psychologically.

Just as it was never nature's intent for man to experience constant physical pain, the same is true emotionally. Man's natural state is positive. Negative emotion serves a very specific purpose—to ensure that people fulfill their basic needs. Chronic negativism blocks the message. Chronic stress and insufficient recovery breed the habitual negativism that undermines our productivity, happiness, and health. Negativism signals unhealthiness, disharmony, and imbalance.

Emotional toughness means the ability to:

- Be flexible, responsive, strong, and resilient under stress
- Sustain a positive emotional state most of the time
- Tune in to the precise recovery message that triggers each negative emotion felt
- Change from a negative emotional state to a positive one quickly

Emotions are biochemical messengers that provide continuous feedback on the balance of stress and recovery in our lives. Maximum *emotional toughness* requires three learnable mind/body attributes:

1. *Mental toughness*—holding tough beliefs and having the habit of thinking tough
2. *Physical toughness*—high physical fitness plus the habit of acting tough
3. *The ability to understand and interpret the meaning of each negative emotion*

Remember, your natural state is positive—a feeling of joy to be living, a feeling of challenge, of confidence. Yet negative emotions are also necessary—they serve vital purposes. Use them, respond to them, but don't block them out!

8

MILITARY

AND SPORT

TOUGHENING

MODELS

The desire to get tougher is an ancient one. At the dawn of history, Sparta was famous for systematically toughening its youth. The Mongol hordes thundering out of Asia during the Middle Ages practiced toughening rituals that only the strongest survived. In pre-Columbian South America the Incas turned boys into men by sending them out empty-handed into the frigid Andes to feed and shelter themselves or die. Throughout the world, few civilizations have flourished unless they employed a toughening system of some kind.

In this chapter we examine two toughening systems that are currently used in our culture.

THE MILITARY TRAINING MODEL

Whether or not we are comfortable with the idea of military power, we have to admit the effectiveness of the military toughening system. It can take undisciplined, immature, unfocused, fearful teenagers and within eight weeks transform most of them into soldiers tough enough to conquer the ultimate fear, the fear of death.

This physical and emotional conversion of acne-scarred teenagers into courageous fighters in so short a time is an astonishing feat. Mankind, of course, has had more than two millennia of experience in training soldiers; the art of getting young men to put their lives on the line has long been a primary concern of the older men who make wars.

Given the age-old success of the military system, I reasoned that studying it would yield many important insights into the toughening process, and many tried and tested methods. That assumption proved true, although getting to the useful things required me to eliminate many features of military training that are useless or even harmful in Toughness Training for Life.

WHY MARCH?

For thousands of years, men marched into battle. Although they're now more likely to ride vehicles into the fighting zone, new recruits still spend many hours marching in formation. Why does the practice of marching remain so central to the making of a soldier?

It's interesting that battles haven't been fought marching since the 18th century. Soldiers don't march on modern battlefields—they run, hide, jump into foxholes, or charge forward. Nobody stays alive very long marching in the face of the enemy. It's clear that in more recent times even when soldiers have still marched *into* battle, that's *not* what they have done during battle. Marching is for *between battles*.

Clearly this regimented practice of walking in a particular way somehow breeds courage, confidence, and decisiveness during battle. To understand how this could be, let's examine the practice more closely. First of all, how do marching soldiers look on the outside? You never see any visible sign of weakness whatsoever. If a soldier is tired, you'll never know it unless he or she totally collapses. No visible fatigue, no sagging shoulders, no negativism, no fear. What you see is total focus, confidence, positive energy, and precision. Every movement is decisive and clean, nothing sloppy or lazy. Every breath is synchronized to exact movement.

Marching prepares soldiers for battle by giving them practice in being decisive, looking strong, and acting confident, regardless of how they feel. It trains discipline, sustained concentration, decisiveness, and poise, all of which are essential elements in conquering fear.

THE MARCH OF CHAMPIONS

It hit me like a ton of bricks—why hadn't I seen it earlier? All great tennis champions have the same walk between points—between their battles—that marching soldiers display. Top, tough competitors show the same focus, confidence, energy, and precision that soldiers do when they walk. No weakness, nothing sloppy, nothing but strength. Tennis champions walk as soldiers march, to bolster courage and control. I've come to refer to it as the *matador walk*.

Practice looking and acting how you want to feel in your performance situations. It pays off for soldiers and athletes. There's a powerful lesson here for all of us.

THE ART OF SOLDIER MAKING

The transition from fearful adolescent to fearless—or at least enormously more confident—warrior occurs in response to imposing the following requirements:

1. A strict code of acting and behaving under stress. This includes:

   - A disciplined way of responding to stress
   - A precise, energetic way of walking, with head and shoulders erect, chin up
   - Quick and decisive response to commands—no hesitation tolerated

2. No visible sign of weakness or negative emotion of any kind in response to stress. The expression of negative emotion is simply not permitted. No matter how you feel, this is the way you act!

3. Regular exposure to high levels of mental, emotional, and phys-

ical training stress to accelerate the toughening process. Obnoxious drill instructors—very tough individuals in the street sense of the word—provide all three kinds of stress.

4. Precise control and regulation of cycles of sleep, eating, drinking, and rest. The regimen includes:

- Up early and to bed early (lights out—no choice)
- Mandatory meals including breakfast—no choice about timing, few choices about foods

5. A rigorous physical fitness program. This essential component of the toughening process involves two elements:

- Aerobic and anaerobic training
- Strength training

6. An enforced schedule of trained recovery. This includes:

- The regimen outlined in item 4 above
- Regularly scheduled R&R
- Enforced cycles of stress followed by enforced cycles of recovery

———— UNDESIRABLE FEATURES OF THE MILITARY TRAINING SYSTEM ————

1. *The stripping of personal identity* and its replacement by group identity (uniforms and short haircuts) is not appropriate in nonmilitary life. Where it does happen—in gangs and cults, primarily—it indicates seriously low levels of self-esteem.
2. *Military values, beliefs, and skills* have little application to civilian life. Many, though not all, of the military skills (for example, close-order drill and heavy weapons use) have no value whatever except in a military career.
3. *Blind adherence to authority* is rarely appropriate outside the military. Military decisions are made by next higher command, not by the individual. In today's fast-paced world we must make our own decisions. In most cases we have no one to look to for direction.

4. *Mental and emotional inflexibility and rigidity* are severely limiting. An influential school of thought holds that flexible thinking should replace the traditional rigidity of the military mind, that even on the battlefield inflexible thinking leads straight to disaster. In any case, rigid military mentalities must shift gears to cope with the subtleties and swift changes of civilian life.

5. *Acquired dislike for physical exercise* is a common result of the pain and boredom of basic training. Although this blind reaction robs some men of any interest in maintaining physical fitness, military service sets a pattern of fitness that many others follow for their entire lives.

THE SPORTS TRAINING MODEL

Getting their athletes to perform with confidence, poise, and precision under pressure is the greatest challenge coaches face. Not surprisingly, they have drawn heavily on military training methods, thus making the sports training model very similar to the military model in many respects. Coaches must train their athletes to control the choking response, the crippling fear of failure. High stakes mean big-time pressure. However, inexperienced competitors often feel enormous pressure at their first events, regardless of how important those competitions may be.

THE GREATEST COMPLIMENT

The ability to perform well under pressure—to stay positive in the face of adversity and maintain feelings of fight and confidence—is called *mental toughness* in the world of sports. The greatest compliment you can pay an athlete is to say, "You are mentally tough."

TRAINING ELEMENTS SUCCESSFUL COACHES HAVE IN COMMON

Great coaches produce athletes who consistently show great courage and poise under pressure. Examples are Vince Lombardi, John Wooden, and James "Doc" Counsilman. Their coaching systems have many common elements, including the three listed here:

1. Strict levels of physical fitness are required, in accordance with their strong belief that mental and emotional fitness are closely linked to physical fitness. They know that a higher level of physical fitness automatically makes an athlete tougher mentally. The overwhelming consensus in sport is that physical fitness leads directly to improved self-confidence and greater emotional strength and resiliency under pressure.
2. They impose a strict code of acting and thinking under pressure. They teach their athletes:

- Never to show weakness on the outside
- Never to talk negatively
- Never to whine or complain
- To think positively
- To look energetic and confident at all times
- To follow a precise way of thinking and acting after making mistakes

3. Strict adherence to rules regarding sleep, alcohol, drugs, and meals is required. Those who violate curfew, alcohol, or drug rules are subject to suspension from the team.
4. Repeated exposure to progressively increasing levels of competitive stress. Toughening does not occur without exposure to stress.

SUMMARY

From the study of military and sport toughening models, a number of common elements become apparent. In both training arenas, the importance of a highly disciplined way of acting and thinking under stress is clearly established. Issues of physical fitness, recovery, the outward projection of strength and confidence, and regular exposure to relatively high levels of training stress are fundamental to successful toughening in both worlds. The transformations in toughness that can occur from the training interventions in the military and sports worlds are often dramatic. Understanding the commonalities provides a strong comparative base for building an effective life-toughening system.

9

GETTING TOUGH

PHYSICALLY

To a weakened person, the approach of more stress poses a threat and gives rise to negative emotions that make it harder—or impossible—to cope with the new stressor. A toughened person, on the other hand, reacts to new or added stress in an emotionally positive way.

Positive reaction to new stress—the challenge response—releases specific hormones that enable the toughened mind and body to cope powerfully with any stressor it has been trained to meet. If the challenge is new, or more intense than previously encountered, the hormones cause the body to respond in an adaptive way that increases its strength, energy, and ability to cope with similar future stressors.

What can we do to speed the learning of this unique response? What kind of physical training works best to strengthen the challenge response? This chapter will answer these questions.

Although emotions are genuine biochemical events, they are not easily accessible. Emotional training for the challenge response occurs in two ways: (1) outside-in (from the muscles inward to the brain), and (2) inside-out (from the brain outward through thinking and perceiving).

Although we don't have direct voluntary control of our emotions, we can exercise considerable control over what we do with our physical bodies as well as the direction and content of our thoughts. Physical toughness and mental toughness together produce emotional toughness, as shown in Figure 9.1. This understanding forms the basis of Toughness Training.

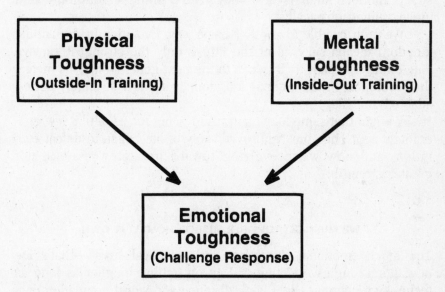

Figure 9.1   Getting Physically and Mentally Tougher Means Automatically Getting Emotionally Tougher

For modern man, it's never been tougher. The sheer volume of stress these days, both business and personal stress, is staggering.

Unlike that experienced by early man, today's stress is emotional, not physical. Hunters and gatherers for millions of years, early man lived a life of rigorous physical activity. Over countless millennia, adaptations of man's cardiovascular, muscular, and energy systems reflected those environmental demands—sudden bursts of physical activity followed by rest and recovery.

Occasional survival conflicts provided nearly all of early man's emotional stress. The scant ten millennia of evolution since mankind began settling down to raise crops have not prepared us to remain motionless for hours on end behind a desk. Nor have they prepared us to consume large quantities of unnatural, nutritionally deficient foods. Even less have they prepared us to confront a nearly endless barrage of emotional stressors. In the language of sport, modern man is seriously overtraining emotionally and undertraining physically.

We're in trouble in another basic way. Evolution in the animal kingdom means survival of the fittest; only the strongest survive long enough to pass their genes to the next generation. This means that evolution in the animal kingdom is toward stronger, better-adapted animals.

We had that same long-term trend going for us until a few generations ago. Then our "improved" way of life began to defeat evolution, and now we're evolving toward greater weakness, not greater strength.

WE MUST GET TOUGHER JUST TO HOLD OUR OWN

Too much emotional stress, too little physical stress—that's life now. It's a tough world that will go on getting tougher as long as technology continues to shrink distance and world population continues to explode. These trends have been accelerating since prehistory; they're not likely to change direction within the lifetime of anyone now breathing earth's air.

In other words, the world is not going to adapt to our emotional needs. This means that if desirable changes are to have a big impact on our lives, we must make them within ourselves. Since the world is getting tougher, we must get tougher just to hold our own—and a lot tougher to move ahead. And we can't get tougher by hiding, denying—or even protecting.

One of the most powerful strategies for getting emotionally tougher is to get *physically* tougher. As you'll come to understand in this chapter, getting physically tougher involves three things:

1. *Improving your physical fitness.* Improved physical fitness not only makes you physically stronger. If done intelligently it also makes you more flexible, responsive, and resilient emotionally.
2. *Looking and acting tougher on the outside.* Acting as if you're tougher helps you feel tougher and believe you are tougher. It's more convincing—to yourself and to anyone else who might be watching—when you *know* you're tougher.
3. *Enhancing physical recovery.* Good nutrition, restful sleep, and powerful oscillation between stress and rest are all essential in building your capability to cope with greater stress and be more productive, healthier, and happier.

THE TOUGHNESS TRAINING MODEL FOR TENNIS

I have spent much of my career exploring ways to intensify tennis players' mental toughness. By far the most effective strategy I have discovered for teaching toughness has been to organize—really to ritualize—what my players think and how they act during the 25-second between-point time.

That time, which can amount to as much as an astonishing four-fifths of a tennis match, had always been thought of as downtime—wasted, nonessential time not worth bothering about.

However, by careful study I learned that what players did and thought *between* points had a major impact on their performance *during* points. Unquestionably, how they handled between-point time often made the difference between winning and losing the match.

What I learned from my studies impelled me to devise a training method to exploit the frequent opportunities to increase performance power that between-point time offers. That training method basically consists of six elements:

1. A highly precise way of thinking and acting under stress
2. Not showing any visible sign of weakness on the outside that could encourage the opponent
3. Projecting IPS (Ideal Performance State) emotions as powerfully as possible during high-stress conditions—particularly high positive energy and confidence
4. Not allowing negative emotions to intrude into the recovery period
5. Highly ritualized preparation routines
6. Maximum physical fitness for maximum recovery

PUTTING THE SYSTEM TO WORK

I've spent countless hours teaching players the most effective behavior they can adopt during the stress of competition. We've worked on how they should walk, hold their heads and shoulders, carry their rackets, and keep their eyes forward and down, among other things.

Parts of my training system parallel military training procedures, although my training method was developed without military influence. I became aware of the similarities only after the model had evolved and been proved effective.

RECOMMENDATIONS FOR ACCELERATING
EMOTIONAL TOUGHNESS

These recommendations are based on the common physical elements for accelerating emotional toughness in the military and athletic models. Figure 9.2 depicts the fundamental importance of recovery and physical toughening in the process of emotional toughening.

- Be certain that you are as well recovered as possible before exposing yourself to great stress.
- Improve your physical fitness.
- Be more precise in the way you look and act under stress—that is, display alertness, energy, and confidence.

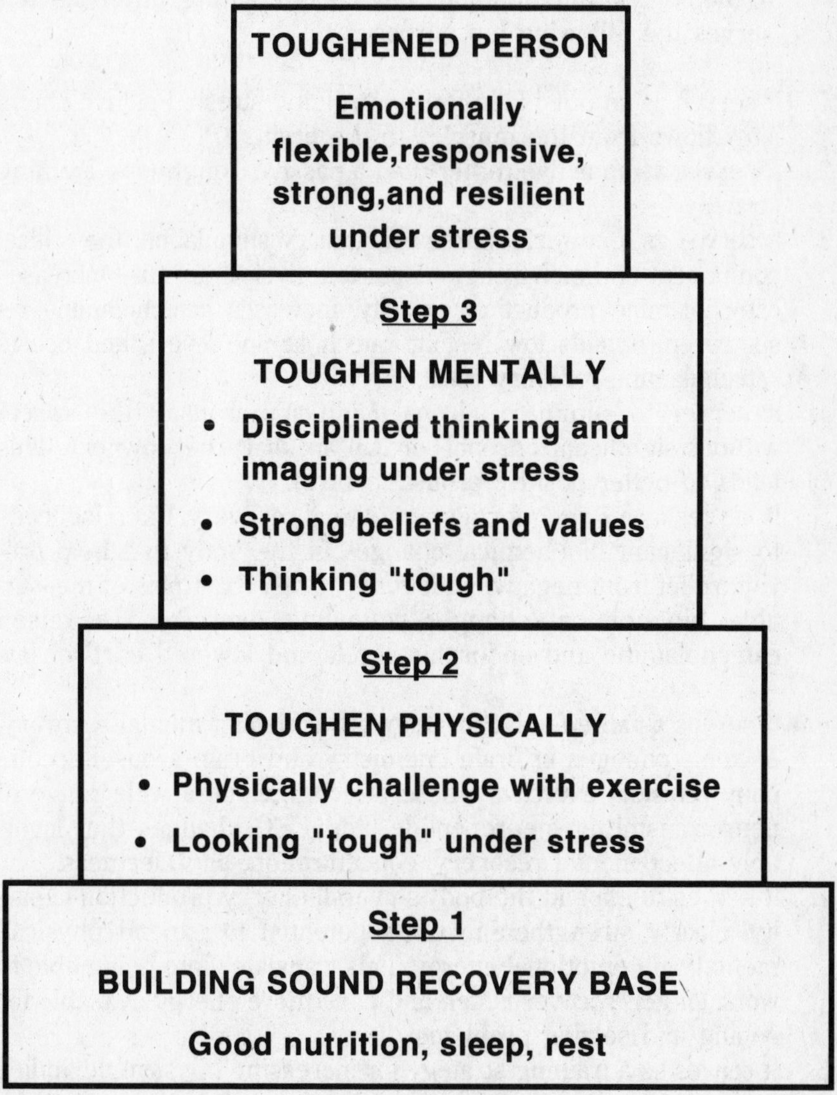

TOUGHENED PERSON

Emotionally flexible, responsive, strong, and resilient under stress

Step 3

TOUGHEN MENTALLY

- **Disciplined thinking and imaging under stress**
- **Strong beliefs and values**
- **Thinking "tough"**

Step 2

TOUGHEN PHYSICALLY

- **Physically challenge with exercise**
- **Looking "tough" under stress**

Step 1

BUILDING SOUND RECOVERY BASE

Good nutrition, sleep, rest

Figure 9.2   The Building Blocks of Toughness Training

WHY PHYSICAL FITNESS?

Why and how does becoming more physically fit lead to improved emotional toughness?

In the context of emotional Toughness Training, physical exercise serves the following ten purposes:

1. It serves as an outside-in form of training stress. Positive chemistry flows from the muscles to the brain.
2. It serves as an active rather than a passive Toughness Training strategy.
3. It serves as a powerful adrenal-medullary stimulation, the critical component in the challenge response. Physical exercise increases catecholamine production capacity, increases catecholamine responsiveness, aids low resting catecholamine levels, and boosts catecholamine recovery rates.
4. It serves to stimulate adrenal-medullary arousal (the upper) without significant adrenal-cortical arousal (the downer). This leads to better positive arousal control.
5. It serves as a strong form of emotional recovery. Exercise leads to significant biochemical changes in the body that help provide relief from negative emotional states. Examples of measurable biochemical changes following exercise are raised catecholamine and endorphin levels and lowered cortisol levels.
6. It serves as an effective strategy for achieving mental recovery, because changes in brain chemistry and brain arousal accompany physical exercise. These effects include a wide range of neurotransmitter, neuropeptide, and EEG changes that favorably affect mental recovery, concentration, and alertness.
7. It serves to expand the body's overall energy production capacity, clearly strengthening one's potential to expend physical, mental, and emotional energy. This translates into being able to work longer, recover faster, and have more energy available for coping and solving problems.
8. It serves as a training strategy for increasing physical flexibility, responsiveness, strength, and resiliency—all markers of physical toughness.
9. It serves to accelerate the learning of recovery mechanisms.

This is particularly the case with interval exercise, in which numerous opportunities exist for training recovery.

10. It serves as an antidepressant strategy. Both aerobic and anaerobic exercise have been shown to have antidepressant effects. Several studies have shown that exercise is a better antidepressant than relaxation and enjoyable activities. Exercise has been shown to be as effective in decreasing depression as many forms of psychotherapy.

───────── **THE MOST EFFECTIVE FORMS OF EXERCISE TO COMBAT** ─────────
───────────────── **DEPRESSION AND BOOST MOTIVATION** ─────────────────

The length and total number of exercise sessions is significant. I have found that the longer individuals were in exercise programs, the more their depression decreased.

There are three possible explanations for this surprising finding:

1. It's known that changes in three neurotransmitters—serotonin, dopamine, and norepinephrine—occur in humans as a result of exercise. Future studies may reveal a precise explanation for the antidepressant effects of those changes.
2. Chronically exercised rats have improved emotionality because the exercise has raised their brain norepinephrine levels.
3. Endorphin increases during exercise have morphine-like qualities that reduce pain and produce a euphoric state. Pert and Bowie found that regularly exercised rats showed an increase in brain endorphin receptor occupancy. While the exact biochemical mechanism is still unknown, it's clear that a connection exists between exercise and reduced pain.

KEY POINT:

ANAEROBIC FORMS OF EXERCISE

DECREASE DEPRESSION AS MUCH AS OR MORE

THAN AEROBIC FORMS DO.

LEARNING THE VITAL SKILL OF LOOKING TOUGH

Why and how does looking and acting tough lead to the improved emotional toughness that improves your physical performance? Although the best answer available from current knowledge oversimplifies an exceedingly complex subject, three points are important:

1. The intimate link between the emotions and the physical body form a transmission network crowded with messages flowing both ways. Two things are clear:

    ■ Feelings lead to changes in how we act and look. For example, smiling at people when greeting them makes us look more friendly. Beyond that, the smile is a friendly action that also predisposes us to treat others in a far more friendly fashion than we would if we had scowled at them.
    ■ How we act and look leads to changes in how we feel.

2. Facial muscle movement can produce measurable autonomic (involuntary) nervous system changes. Researchers Paul Ekman, Robert Levenson, and Wallace Friesen at the University of California's School of Medicine demonstrated that contraction of facial muscles in the direction of surprise, disgust, sadness, anger, fear, and happiness stimulated emotion—specific autonomic activity. For example, looking angry actually triggers the chemical basis of anger. In other words, making a mad face—that is, simply moving the facial muscles to form the expression of anger—is enough to start the characteristic blood chemistry of anger moving.

3. The autonomic responses (heart rate, finger temperature, skin resistance, and muscle tension) were similar whether subjects

were actually reliving past experiences using imagery, or simply moving their facial muscles in the desired direction. This finding provides a clear example of how closely linked certain muscles are to emotion.

————————— THE POWER OF "AS IF" —————————

- How you walk, how you carry your head and shoulders, and the expression on your face can stimulate emotion-specific responses.
- Acting *as if* you feel a particular way can get the chemistry moving in that direction.
- Looking calm, challenged, energetic, and confident in a stressful situation may begin as a faked look. However, that faked look can quickly lead to a genuine emotion—that is, to a specific biochemical response that has a very positive effect on performance.
- Acting *as if* is a trained response—the more you do it, the better you'll be at making it work.

THE FIRST RULE OF TOUGHNESS:

PROJECT TO THE WORLD OUTSIDE YOUR

SKIN WHAT YOU WANT TO FEEL INSIDE.

————————— COCKINESS IN LIFE AND SPORT —————————

To bolster confidence and hide their insecurities, many children learn to project cockiness at an early age. Typically these adaptations to life's pressures intensify in adolescence and begin disappearing in adulthood.

Many adults become overly concerned that cockiness can lead to disaster. It often does, especially cockiness that isn't backed by competence, determination, and physical fitness.

However, in both small endeavors and large undertakings, far more people fail because they lack confidence than because they lack competence or fitness. Where does determination come into it? Determination often dies in people who lack confidence.

In other words, people beat themselves more than difficulties or opponents do. Both in sport and in life, this happens all too often to the nontough.

TOUGHNESS TRAINING TIP:

LOOKING THE WAY YOU FEEL ENHANCES

YOUR CURRENT FEELING. IF YOU DON'T

LIKE YOUR CURRENT EMOTIONAL STATE,

CHANGE THE WAY YOU LOOK.

GAINING MORE CONTROL OF HOW YOU ACT AND LOOK

Developing a strict code for how you act and look under stress gives you a large degree of control of your stress response. Following that code consistently increases your control of negative arousal so that you can better avoid the feelings of fear, frustration, and failure that cause despair, defeat, and disaster.

From Michael Jordan to Wayne Gretsky in sport and from Lee Iacocca to Ross Perot in business, top performers project strong, powerful images when they perform under stress.

WHY BE WELL RECOVERED?

Why is being well recovered so important to emotional toughness?

Because no matter how tough you are, if your body can no longer produce sufficient energy, the emotional strength essential to success soon becomes impossible. Everyone stops fighting when blood sugar levels drop to a certain point. As Vince Lombardi said so aptly, "Fatigue makes cowards of us all."

This reality is enormously more evident in sport than in life because athletic contests, besides being structured for maximum visibility, are conducted according to rigid rules concerning time and space and match opponents of similar abilities. Competition in life is comparatively unstructured, is less visible, is often conducted under few or no rules regarding time and space, and frequently throws opponents of vastly different capabilities and resources against each other.

Although individual cases of poor recovery are not as obvious in life as they are in sport, this effect is no less vital in ordinary living. You may not engage in athletic competition, but the effects of poor recovery apply just as much to you as they do to every professional athlete. In the remainder of this section, see yourself standing in the athlete's shoes.

Here are three essentials of good physical recovery:

1. *Choose your recovery habits with care.* Undisciplined athletes who don't follow sensible rules regarding sleep, diet, and drugs are the most likely to crack under pressure. In other words, they collapse first. Since most contests in life as in sport are to some degree endurance tests, this means that undisciplined athletes always lose to disciplined athletes of the same ability. The same is true in any kind of competition in business or in life.
2. *Recover before taking on a new stressor.* One of the most important steps you can take to be emotionally tough in a given situation is to be physically well recovered before you encounter another bout of stress.
3. *Defend yourself against low blood sugar.* Guard against letting your blood sugar level bottom out between meals. People on the three-square-meals-a-day nutrition system often have this problem; people who skip breakfast almost always are severely weakened by it.

HOW TO AVOID LOW BLOOD SUGAR

The need to avoid low blood sugar between meals all too often is met by consuming food or drink laced with simple sugar. Unfortunately the items most often consumed during work breaks— cookies, doughnuts, candy bars, and soft drinks—do a terrific job of defeating recovery by spiking blood sugar levels.

Few people realize that cookies, candy, ice cream, and soft drinks, or coffee with a spoonful of sugar will push their blood sugar levels so far down they feel exhausted. Common sense tells you that taking in sugar will raise your blood sugar level, not drop it. And that's exactly what happens—at first.

All the popular snacks mentioned above contain simple sugars that reach the bloodstream very quickly—especially from the typical coffee-breaker's empty stomach. The quick jolt of sugar causes the pancreas to release so much insulin that the body's blood sugar level is driven down. Often it falls well below what it was before the sugar was swallowed.

The usual scenario runs like this. On most days, Sharon, a typical office worker who has scanty breakfasts or skips them entirely, feels a little trembly with hunger as the hands of the office clock slowly crawl toward her 10:30 morning break.

Every day at 10:30 exactly, Sharon hurries down the hall to the employee cafeteria. There she usually has two or three doughnuts (she likes the glazed sugar ones) and drinks a cup of coffee after stirring in two spoonfuls of sugar. If she has time, she drinks a second cup of coffee.

At the beginning of the break, Sharon often feels glum, but within minutes her blood sugar has soared and, feeling vivacious, she happily chatters with her fellow office workers. All too soon the break is over and Sharon heads back to her desk.

Feeling peppy as she sits down, Sharon tackles her work with enthusiasm. But within 20 to 30 minutes her energy vanishes, she decides she hates her job, and she starts watching the clock again. Sharon hopes she can keep her production up until the lunch break and wonders why she feels so rotten.

Sharon feels bad because the sugary doughnuts spiked her blood sugar level, giving her a few minutes of high spirits that she attributed to being on a break with her friends. However, returning to work had little to do with her sudden fatigue. That happened because her pancreas, reacting to the sudden rise in her blood sugar level, released enough insulin to control the problem. The caffeine in the coffee she drank did nothing to slow the process.

The problem is that refined sugar is a recent invention; no human being ever tasted it until a few hundred years ago. Although we rely on the complex sugars found in natural foods for energy and cope easily with their slower conversion into blood sugar, refined sugar still hits us too hard too fast.

─────────── **THE *TOUGH*™ WAFER** ───────────

The absence of a perfect between-meals snack is precisely why I petitioned Solaray to produce the *Tough*™ line of energy/recovery products. I felt there was a complete absence of convenient between-meals snacks that take up little space, can be quickly and easily consumed, have minimal spoilage problems, and don't create a lot of litter. Without success, I searched long and hard for products that would provide energy for people without pounding them with simple sugars, fat, or preservatives. Eventually it became clear that I'd have to develop the product myself.

Tough™ brand wafers* make it easier for athletes, schoolchildren, and executives to meet their energy recovery needs—specifically, to do a better job of:

- Meeting carbohydrate intake requirements
- Stabilizing blood sugar
- Restoring muscle glycogen and liver glycogen levels

BECOMING MORE FIT

Maintaining or improving physical fitness prevents muscle degeneration caused by inactivity, weight gain, or the aging process. Exercise is a full partner with intelligent eating habits in every weight loss program that succeeds; it's also the only way of slowing the aging process that works.

However, muscle degeneration is not exclusive to the elderly, by any means—it can strike at any age. Anyone who is not physically active—even a child—can suffer muscle degeneration. Many of today's young snack-munching TV-watchers are well into a spiral of deteriorating health. Low physical activity adds to weight gain caused by a bad diet, and the weight gain makes physical activity even less attractive. When this less exercise/more weight/less exercise spiral begins in early childhood, it often accelerates steadily

*Information regarding the Tough™ product line is available from the Loehr-Groppel/ Saddlebrook Sport Science Center in Wesley Chapel, Florida.

as time passes. Many fifth-grade fatties are obese by thirty and dead by fifty.

HOW PHYSICAL FITNESS PAYS OFF

Enhancing your physical fitness pays off in four fundamental ways:

1. Improved physical flexibility
2. Improved physical responsiveness
3. Improved physical strength
4. Improved physical resiliency

Let's examine each of these four ways in detail.

IMPROVING YOUR PHYSICAL FLEXIBILITY

Physical flexibility increases in response to a program of progressively stretching muscles to move through their full range of motion. To avoid injuring muscles and joints—and becoming stiffer than before—this must be done gently and painlessly without bouncing.

Many people move more easily and can exercise more with less pain after improving flexibility in the following areas: low back, neck, hamstring, and shoulder.

Two of the most common complaints people have today are low back pain and neck pain. Both are often related to poor muscle flexibility in those areas.

Recommended Procedures
Specific flexibility exercises are presented later in this chapter. The following are general principles of such exercises.

1. *Warm up first.* Stretching should always come *after* a warm-up period. The importance of warming up before you start stretching can't be overemphasized. Raise your body temperature by running or jogging in place to make your muscles and tendons more pliable.
2. *Stretch at least four times a week.* Five times a week is better.

The stretching program recommended later in this chapter takes seven to ten minutes.

3. *Use static stretching.* This involves holding the stretch for about ten seconds and then relaxing.
4. *Don't bounce as you stretch.* Bouncing increases the risk of injury.
5. *Don't force the stretch.* Go as far as is comfortable and then hold the stretch.

──────────── **IMPROVING YOUR PHYSICAL RESPONSIVENESS** ────────────

Physical responsiveness develops with muscle use and diminishes with disuse. Use it or lose it.

Accident or disease aside, there are three basic causes of declining muscle responsiveness: lack of activity, weight gain, and aging. The last one can be slowed by controlling the first two.

Many physically inactive elderly people have great difficulty driving because their muscles have become nonresponsive. To a considerable degree this can be reversed by a program of gradually increasing exercise in as many different ways as possible. The following recommended procedures, however, apply to all ages.

Recommended Procedures

1. *Vary your exercise.* Engage in as wide a variety of exercise as possible. The more you challenge your cardiovascular and muscular systems in different ways, the more responsive they become. Participate in both aerobic and anaerobic activities if possible. Walking, running, swimming, calisthenics, free weights, weight machines, cycling, and stretching are basic methods, some of which are always available.
2. *Get into fun sports in a big way.* Muscular responsiveness is a key element in every physical sport you can name. Choose the safest and most challenging ones you are capable of doing well enough to enjoy. If your physical condition permits, choose mountain or rock climbing, fly-fishing or surf fishing, downhill or cross-country skiing, handball or Ping-Pong, tennis or badminton, water-skiing or wind-surfing. There are many other en-

joyable physical activities, and your area is ideal for some or
most of them.
3. *Take the active route whenever you can.* Use the elevator less
and the stairs more; instead of driving, cycle or walk whenever
it's reasonable; use a push lawnmower instead of a powered
one; prefer active recreations such as dancing to passive ones
such as moviegoing.

--------------- **IMPROVING YOUR PHYSICAL STRENGTH** ---------------

Greater physical strength is developed by exposing muscles to progressively greater resistance over time. Two key points must be
observed:

1. The overload must be increased gradually in order for adaptation to occur.
2. The load must challenge the muscle but not be so great as to
break it down.

Recommended Procedures

1. *Follow a written schedule.* Control your strength-building program by using a written schedule of weights, sets, and reps
(repetitions).
2. *Go for ten repetitions.* Start with a weight you can lift ten times
before exhaustion. This is called a ten-repetition maximum (10
RM).
3. *Aim for the best strength gain.* For optimal strength development, exercise in sets of five to seven repetitions for each
weight-lifting exercise. Take two or three minutes to rest between sets.
4. *Maintain the challenge.* Once you can perform the scheduled
number of repetitions easily, you're ready to increase the
weight. Increases of five to ten pounds are usually appropriate
for the large muscles of the legs; use increases of five pounds
or less for most other smaller muscles.
5. *Take your pick.* Weight machines, free weights, and rubber
tubing can all be used to build strength. The choice is really a
matter of convenience, cost, and preference.

GOOD NEWS!

RESEARCH CONFIRMS THAT WEIGHT LIFTING EXTENDS FUNCTIONAL LIFE. THE CAPACITY OF OLDER PEOPLE TO BENEFIT FROM WEIGHT TRAINING PROGRAMS HAS NOW BEEN FIRMLY ESTABLISHED.

AFTER THE AGE OF 30, 10 PERCENT OF MUSCLE MASS IS LOST EVERY DECADE. HOWEVER, THIS CAN BE REVERSED WITH WEIGHT TRAINING. THE ELDERLY CAN DOUBLE THEIR REPETITION MAXIMUM (THE AMOUNT OF WEIGHT THEY CAN LIFT IN A GIVEN EXERCISE) IN 12 WEEKS. EVEN FRAIL PEOPLE IN THEIR NINETIES HAVE GAINED STRENGTH AND IMPROVED THEIR MOBILITY THROUGH A CAREFULLY MONITORED COURSE OF WEIGHT LIFTING.

CLEARLY, THE BENEFITS OF STRENGTH TRAINING ARE NOT LIMITED TO YOUTH.

IMPROVING YOUR PHYSICAL RESILIENCY

Physical resiliency refers to how fast a person recovers from physical stress. Recovery speed between sets is an excellent measure of fitness; it improves in response to intermittent and progressively increasing episodes of physical stress.

Faster muscular and cardiovascular recovery can be achieved with both steady-state and interval exercise. However, proof of the superiority of interval exercise in recovery training is accumulating rapidly.

It seems logical that the best way to train for faster recovery would be through exposure to repeated recovery opportunities. This is precisely what happens in interval exercise.

Recovery can be trained (speeded up) in either of two ways: by progressively decreasing recovery time between cycles of stress, or by increasing the volume of stress and keeping recovery time the same.

Muscle resiliency is achieved by progressively stressing (loading) the muscle and controlling the recovery time between sets using free weights, weight machines, spring-loaded devices, or your equipment of choice.

Cardiovascular resiliency is achieved by progressively stressing the heart and lungs and controlling the recovery time between intervals—that is, by varying the intensity of the exercise on fast-slow-fast-slow cycles.

MORE GOOD NEWS!

JUST LIKE MUSCLES, THE BRAIN ADAPTS TO A CONSISTENT EXERCISE REGIME. RESEARCH AT THE UNIVERSITY OF ILLINOIS BY WILLIAM GREENOUGH DETERMINED THAT MICE THAT WERE EXERCISED ON TREADMILLS AND TAUGHT A BALANCING TASK HAD MORE BRAIN CONNECTIONS AND BLOOD VESSELS THAN MICE THAT GOT SIGNIFICANTLY LESS EXERCISE.

GREENOUGH'S WORK INDICATES THAT THE BRAIN RESPONDS TO PHYSICAL EXERCISE MUCH AS ANY MUSCLE DOES. IF HE'S RIGHT, COULD IT BE THAT EXERCISING MAY ACTUALLY MAKE YOU SMARTER?

THE UNIVERSITY OF UTAH'S ROBERT DUSTMAN INVESTIGATED THE ELECTRICAL BRAIN ACTIVITY OF ELDERLY PEOPLE. DUSTMAN COMPARED AN ATHLETIC GROUP TO A SEDENTARY GROUP. THE ATHLETIC GROUP'S BRAIN WAVES RESEMBLED THOSE OF YOUNGER PEOPLE; THE SEDENTARY GROUP'S DID NOT. IN OTHER WORDS, EXERCISING KEEPS YOU YOUNG.

PHYSICAL FITNESS PRIORITIES FOR LIFE TOUGHENING

Before you start any exercise program, get a medical examination.

PRIORITY #1: STRENGTHEN STOMACH MUSCLES

The muscles of the stomach, the abdominals and obliques, are the basis of all strength. Yet they are the weakest link for most people. Strong stomach muscles protect the low back from injury. This makes strengthening them the underpinning for all further physical toughening. Stronger abdominal muscles build the foundation for breathing during cardiorespiratory workouts.

Recommended Exercise
Strengthen the stomach muscles with bent-knee curl-ups.

- Lie on your back on a soft surface with your knees raised toward your chest and your hands clasped behind your head. Rise up slowly and touch your left elbow to your right knee and slowly return your back to the floor. Next rise up and touch your right elbow to your left knee and return to the floor. One repetition consists of a touch to each knee. Do the curl-up slowly without pulling your head and neck forward with your hands.
- Begin with sets of five and gradually work toward sets of 25 over several weeks.

GOAL: 200 repetitions a day in sets of 25, five days a week.

───────── PRIORITY #2: CHALLENGE HEART AND LUNGS ─────────

Improving cardiorespiratory fitness develops a more efficient energy production system and increases your endurance.

Recommended Exercises
Use a wide variety of challenges to your heart and lungs. Rotate your heart and lung challenges among such exercises as walking, cycling, swimming, and jogging.

- Use a heart rate monitor on all heart and lung challenge exercises.
- Eighty percent of your workout should be up and down cycles (interval training) within your aerobic zone. Your aerobic zone is 65 to 80% of your estimated maximum heart rate. Compute your estimated maximum heart rate by subtracting your age from 220.
- Twenty percent of your workout should be in cycles above and below your aerobic zone.
- Those unaccustomed to exercise should first have a medical ex-

amination, and then avoid exceeding their aerobic zone for their first two months of regular exercise.

- Use interval training instead of continuous exercise. Interval training—as opposed to steady-state training—is more in keeping with life stress.

GOAL: To exercise three or four days a week for a minimum of 20 minutes a day.

KEY POINT:

FOR TOUGHNESS TRAINING PURPOSES, THE

IDEAL LENGTH OF AN EXERCISE PERIOD

IS BETWEEN 20 AND 30 MINUTES.

INTERVAL VS. STEADY-STATE TRAINING

We will compare interval training to the more common steady-state method in considerable detail because recent research shows that interval exercise is superior. First let's explain what the terms mean.

Steady-state exercise has little or no variation in speed or stress level throughout the exercise session. This is low-tech exercise, done the way it's been done since the ancient Greeks trained for the original Olympics. See Figure 9.3.

Interval exercise pulsates. It speeds up and slows down. This is high-tech exercise when it's closely monitored to keep the exerciser's heartbeat within his or her best training range. This makes interval exercise ideal for individuals with cardiovascular problems who are exercising with a doctor's approval. See Figure 9.4.

Interval exercise can be done on a low-tech basis—but this should be done only by people who are physically fit and have no cardiovascular concerns. All you need is a wristwatch or wall clock that shows the seconds. From time to time as you exercise, check your pulse for six seconds and add a zero to get your heart rate per minute.

Try this on your resting heart rate of about 60. In six seconds

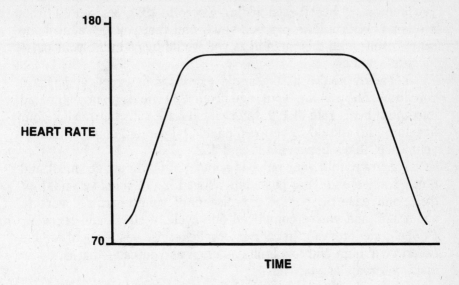

Figure 9.3   Steady-State Aerobic Exercise

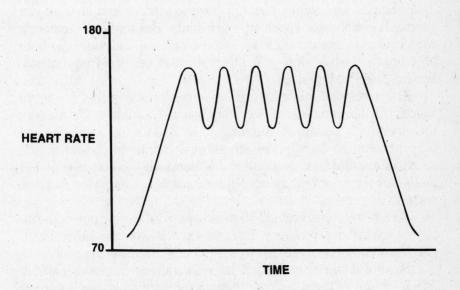

Figure 9.4   Interval Aerobic Exercise

you'll count six heartbeats; adding a zero to six gives you 60 beats a second. With a little practice you'll find that you get almost the same results with this method as you would by counting your pulse for a full minute.

Let's say you're a 30-year-old exerciser in excellent physical condition. Subtracting your age from 220 yields your estimated maximum heart rate of 190. Interval exercise calls for moving your heart rate up and down between 65 and 80 percent of maximum. In your case, that's between 124 and 152.

Warm up until your pulse is about 124 (12 in six seconds) and then exercise until your pulse hits about 152 (15 in six seconds). At that point ease off on the exercise until your heart recovers to about 124, and you've completed one cycle of stress and recovery ("done" one interval). In each interval exercise session, pulsate between your high and low limits as often as you can—that is, do as many intervals as you can.

Obviously it's easier to do intervals with a chest monitor that gives you instant readout. Actually, since the monitors average your pulse, they are about five seconds behind. This means that for maximum benefit and safety, you still have to anticipate a little as you approach either your upper or lower limits. But high-tech intervals with a monitor are certainly far more efficient—and more likely to be continued—than low-tech intervals that require frequent six-second pulse-taking stops.

The stress of interval exercise comes in waves that are more specific to the demands of everyday living. Nothing in life mirrors the stress of a marathon. Running 15 to 20 miles at a steady pace prepares you to handle the stress of a marathon; however, life stress is not like that. Nothing in life demands a heart rate of 140 to 160 for three or four hours without a break. Life stress is *intermittent.*

Steady-state exercise for 30 minutes provides only one opportunity to experience recovery. Interval exercise, on the other hand, provides many opportunities to experience and train recovery.

Several studies report that interval training improves aerobic fitness. Some of them indicate that strength training also improves aerobic capacity.

University of Massachusetts researcher Ann Ward studied the effect of interval vs. continuous (steady-state) exercise on oxygen intake, which is an excellent measure of cardiovascular fitness. She compared two groups covering the same mileage on a 12-minute stationary bike exercise routine.

Both groups used the same frequency of training (three days a week), but one group did interval training (fast-slow, fast-slow) and the other group did steady-state exercise the entire time. Surprisingly, the interval-training group increased their oxygen intake by 11 percent during the 12 weeks of training while the steady-state exercisers' oxygen intake remained the same.

A related study conducted by Arlette Perry at the University of Miami produced similar results. Perry found that over a 12-week training period, interval training produced an 18 percent increase in cardiovascular endurance and steady-state training produced only an 8 percent increase.

Doing intervals allows you to work both the aerobic and anaerobic energy systems.

Exercising aerobically generally means working at between 65 percent and 80 percent of your maximum heart rate, as discussed earlier. Aerobic means "with oxygen"; exercising aerobically means exercising without running out of breath.

Suppose you are 40 years old. If when you exercise you maintain your heart rate between 117 and 144, you challenge your cardiovascular system in a way that does not exceed your body's capacity to supply sufficient oxygen to meet the energy needs. By using a heart rate monitor, you can do intervals between 117 and 144, meet the aerobic requirements, and also stimulate anaerobic activity.

Exercising anaerobically means challenging the cardiovascular system in a way that exceeds the body's capacity to supply sufficient oxygen to meet the energy demands. It's exercising hard enough to run yourself out of breath. For example, a 100-yard dash that leaves you panting is anaerobic; a six-kilometer run at a pace within your conditioned running capacity that doesn't leave you panting is aerobic.

Obviously, exercise that's severe enough will quickly exhaust even the most physically fit, and would be extremely dangerous for a nonexerciser or anyone who has heart, lung, or circulation problems.

By training in intervals within your aerobic band—a heart rate of 117 to 144 if you are the 40-year-old we have been discussing—you are able to repeatedly challenge your anaerobic system as you increase from 117 to 144. You also stimulate small waves of recovery when you decrease intensity from 144 to 117. The interval type of exercise has the advantage of simultaneously:

- Challenging the aerobic energy system
- Challenging the anaerobic energy system
- Providing many opportunities for training recovery

WHY INTERVAL TRAINING IS PREFERABLE TO CONTINUOUS TRAINING

If flexibility, responsiveness, strength, and resiliency are the features of a healthy cardiovascular system, then we must prefer an interval-type exercise plan to continuous exercise. Let's compare a nonexerciser, a steady-state marathon runner, and someone who trains using interval exercise—all of them 40 years old.

NONEXERCISER WHO IS 40 YEARS OLD

Heart flexibility: His resting heart rate is 80, and his formula maximum is 180 (220 less 40). Flexibility range is 100.

Responsiveness: Poor. As reflected in heart rate data, nonexerciser constantly overresponds and underresponds to doses of physical stress.

Strength: Poor. Incapable of effectively handling high doses of physical stress.

Resiliency: Poor. Slow recovery times following doses of physical stress.

MARATHON RUNNER WHO IS 40 YEARS OLD

Runs between 8 and 20 miles a day using steady-state, continuous training methods. The prolonged linear cycles of physical stress have caused the usual highly specific cardiovascular adaptations that all distance runners acquire.

Heart flexibility: Resting heart rate of 42, but has difficulty achieving his estimated maximum heart rate of 180. Functional range is 42 to approximately 170; flexibility range is thus 128.

Responsiveness: Long linear cycles of physical stress do not lead to maximum responsiveness to physical or emotional stressors. Chronic stress (linear) leads to reduced sensitivity.

Strength: Capable of handling very high doses of physical stress effectively, but readily achievable maximum cardiac output in response to physical stress is reduced.

Resiliency: Marathon training results in excellent recovery speed, particularly in activities similar to those used in training.

INTERVAL EXERCISER WHO IS 40 YEARS OLD

Exercises 30 to 60 minutes a day using a wide variety of training exercises, including walking, biking, swimming, running, and tennis. Trains using intervals rather than continuous methods. Does approximately 80 percent of his training doing intervals within his aerobic band (117–144). Does the remaining 20 percent using intervals below and above the aerobic training zone.

Heart flexibility: His resting heart rate is 50. Since he can readily achieve his estimated maximum heart rate of 180 if necessary, his functional range is 130.

Responsiveness: Interval training clearly enhances sensitivity and responsiveness of the cardiovascular system to physical stress. Interval exercise trains the heart and lungs to quickly respond to and recover from sudden increases in work output.

Strength: Capable of a powerful cardiovascular response to physical stress. Able to readily achieve estimated maximum heart rates.

Resiliency: Interval training results in maximum recovery speed.

PRIORITY #3: INCREASE GENERAL MUSCLE STRENGTH

Use free weights, machines, flexible rubber tubing, or your own body resistance (as in push-ups). Challenge alternate muscle groups on alternate days. For example, challenge the upper body on Mondays, Wednesdays, and Fridays, and the lower body on Tuesdays, Thursdays, and Saturdays.

Muscle Groups to Be Toughened
- Abdominal muscles (covered in Priority #1)
- Large muscles of the legs
- Large muscles of the back
- Chest muscles
- Arm and shoulder muscles

Recommended Repetitions
For maximum strength training purposes, 5 to 7 RM for three sets is recommended with two to five minutes of recovery between sets. Once you can perform the exercise ten times, increase the weight by five to ten pounds.

Determining Your Starting Lift Weight
When starting a program the safest way to determine how much weight you should lift is to use the ten-repetition test. If you can perform the exercise more than ten times, increase the weight by five pounds, or by 5 to 10 percent of the total weight.

It is common to use the maximum amount of weight one can perform in a single repetition (called a one-repetition maximum of 1 RM) to determine how much weight should be used for the sets. However, this increases the risk of injury, which is greatest when one attempts maximal contraction.

Some Tips
- Getting certified supervision is smart. When starting a free weight or machine strength training program, always begin with supervision from a properly trained and certified professional. Learning proper lifting and training techniques is critical to ensure safety and progress.
- Don't cheat yourself. There are ways to cheat on many exercises—ways to lift a little more weight using improper lifting movements. However, cheating exercisers only cheat themselves, because the improper movements don't properly stress the desired muscles.
- Don't skip warm-up. Always begin your strength training with proper warm-up exercises to prevent injury.

PRIORITY #4: INJURY PREVENTION THROUGH FLEXIBILITY TRAINING AND SPECIFIC STRENGTHENING OF HIGH-RISK AREAS

Muscle flexibility plays a critical role in any injury prevention program. The following stretching program is recommended for general life toughening.

GOAL: Do your stretch routine at least five times a week. Stretching every day is better.

RECOMMENDED GENERAL STRETCHING PROGRAM

Always begin your stretching routine with a warm-up drill that will make your muscles and tendons more pliable.

Stretch #1
(Calf Stretch)
Perform twice for 20 seconds each leg.

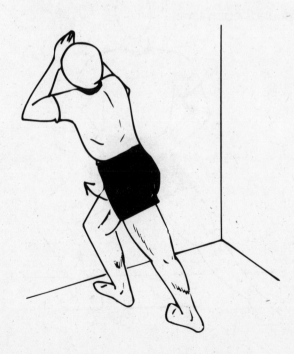

Stretch #2
(Hip and Quads Stretch)
Perform twice for 20 seconds each leg.

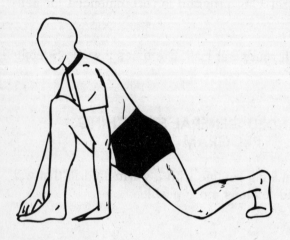

Stretch #3
(Groin Stretch)
Perform twice for 20 seconds each time.

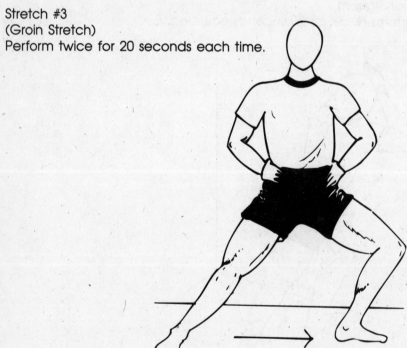

Stretch #4
(Hamstring Stretch)
Perform twice for 20 seconds each time.

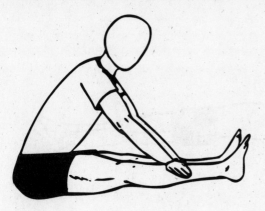

Stretch #5
(Low Back and Hip Stretch)
Perform twice for 20 seconds each leg and 20 seconds for both
legs.

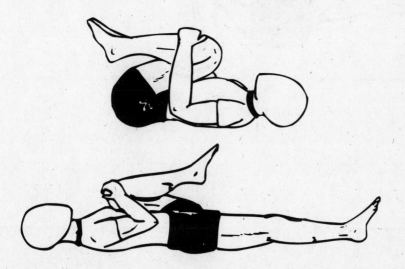

Stretch #6
(Abdominal Stretch)
Perform twice for 20 seconds each time.

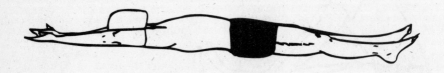

Stretch #7
(Low Back and Hip Stretch)
Perform twice for 20 seconds each side.

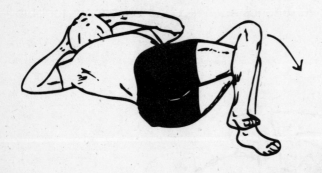

Stretch #8
(Shoulder and Back Stretch)
Perform twice for 20 seconds each time.

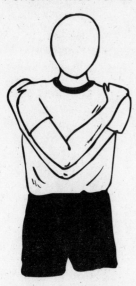

Stretch #9
(Triceps Stretch)
Perform twice for 20 seconds each arm.

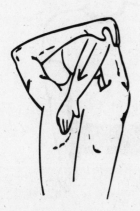

Stretch #10
(Shoulder Stretch)
Perform twice for 20 seconds each arm.

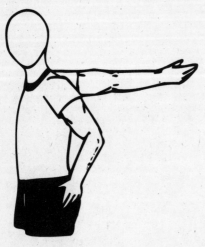

Stretch #11
(Neck Stretch)
Perform twice for 20 seconds each side.

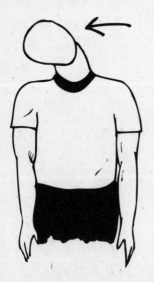 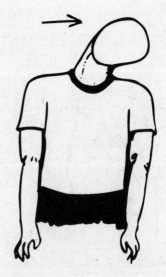

Stretch #12
(Arm and Side Stretch)
Perform both stretching exercises for 20 seconds each side.

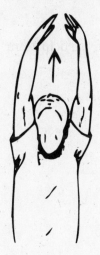
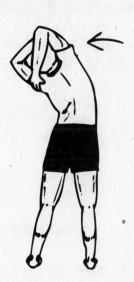

PROTECT YOURSELF FROM INJURY

The best way to protect your most susceptible and vulnerable areas from injury is to strengthen the muscles surrounding those areas. For most people, ankles, knees, shoulders, and elbows are the most vulnerable areas. Every sports participant owes these areas special attention in the form of strengthening exercises. However, if you know you have weak ankles or knees, it means that you are more prone to injury there. In such a case, be sure to protect yourself by doing strength training exercises targeted to your particular weaknesses. Begin challenging the weakened areas with progressive doses of stress immediately. Consult with a physical therapist or conditioning specialist to design the best training exercises for you, especially if you have any health or disability problem, haven't exercised regularly in the last two years, or are over 40.

Participating in sports places special demands on the body,

and these should be considered as part of your injury prevention program. For most participants, the high-risk areas are:

- Skiing and basketball: knees and ankles
- Tennis and golf: shoulders, back, and elbows

Strengthen your weaknesses so you can continue to participate in your chosen sport—for a lifetime!

TOUGHNESS TIP:

DON'T WAIT UNTIL YOU'RE INJURED

AGAIN TO START TOUGHENING. LAUNCH

YOUR PROGRAM TODAY.

FINAL EXERCISE GUIDELINES

- Prior to beginning an exercise program, have a thorough medical exam.
- Start slowly.
- Get started with professional supervision, particularly in the area of weight training.
- Make it fun.
- Question the coaching expertise of anybody who says, "No gain without pain." However, we must distinguish between the mild and pleasant burning sensation one gets in a muscle that's stressed enough to cause it to toughen, and the tearing pain of injury or the sharp pain of a stretch too far.
- Pain is *not* part of the program, but fun is!
- Use a heart rate monitor at all times during exercise and stay within your exercise guidelines. For accuracy, monitors that use *chest* sensors are recommended (belt around the chest). Although these monitors usually have excellent accuracy, they can produce erroneous readings. Always monitor your perceived exertion to confirm the results—in other words, don't blindly rely on the monitor. If you have further questions regarding a heart rate monitor, consult an exercise specialist or your physician.

- Use the widest variety of exercise possible. This will prevent boredom and lead to a higher level of functional fitness.
- Use low-impact, soft-surface exercise as much as possible to protect the body from shock and pounding. Examples are running on grass, cycling, cross-country-skiing simulators, and rebound exercise.
- As much as possible, use interval training rather than continuous, steady-state training methods.
- Increase your training loads gradually over time.
- Use low-risk sports like tennis to achieve your life toughening goals.
- The interval nature of tennis makes it an ideal sport for life toughening. Between-point time in recreational tennis provides frequent, low-risk opportunities to practice your toughening skills: the confident manner and walk, resting your eyes on the racket, concentration, and especially keeping up a constant flow of positive images and thoughts that will prevent any negative emotion from hurting your performance.
- Follow a consistent program both to maintain and to improve your fitness.

10

GETTING

TOUGH

MENTALLY

Emotion rules our lives. Most of the decisions we make are emotional—after our emotions have decided, we use our heads to come up with logical reasons that justify our often impulsive decisions and actions. This is especially true in our relationships—in all our dealings with other people.

Life, law, and reality make no allowances for emotion's rule. We suffer the consequences of our emotional impulses if they're unfavorable, and reap the benefits if they're on target. Yes, emotion rules our lives, yet emotion doesn't think, doesn't reason, doesn't weigh alternatives—and in fact can't.

At its worst, emotion rules with panic and rage; at its best, with sublime poise and confidence—the Ideal Performance State. But most of the time we live between those extremes, where we can and must consciously direct our primitive limbic brain with our thinking cortex.

It takes mental toughness to control our emotions. In fact, the key to all success is having—and using—enough mental toughness to control our emotions and thus our actions.

What changes or adaptations can we make *mentally* that will help us gain more control *emotionally*? We have to do it mentally because we can't directly reach our emotions.

Mental training—that is, mental *toughening*—is inside-out training. It starts inside the brain and moves outward to the body.

We think in words and images (visualization). We have almost total control over both, although few of us have developed the ability to visualize positive images as quickly and powerfully as we easily could. Curiously enough, we all seem to have strong natural capabilities to conjure up negative images, probably because this facility is more strongly driven by emotion. And therein lies the key to developing our ability to visualize positive images.

KEY POINT:

DEVELOP YOUR ABILITY TO VISUALIZE

POSITIVE IMAGES BY LOADING THEM WITH

POSITIVE EMOTION.

- What changes can be made in the way we think and visualize that will enable us to more readily access Ideal Performance State emotions, positive feelings states, and positive arousal?
  - We can remember and mentally intensify scenes in which we performed superlatively.
  - We can remember and mentally intensify the emotions we felt when we performed superlatively.
- Is there a connection between how and what we think and our moment-to-moment emotional state?
- Can we train mentally to experience empowered emotional states more often?

Clearly, the answer to the latter two questions is *yes!*

APPLIED INSIDE-OUT MENTAL TRAINING

Much of my work with athletes over the past 18 years has been inside-out mental training. This involves training athletes how to think tough so they can feel tough in competition. In the course of this work, I've developed a great respect for the delicate connection between thought and emotion.

Dramatic examples of a single thought's power abound in golf. The images or thoughts you hold during your golf swing largely determine the outcome of the shot. Merely shifting your attention to various parts of your body as you swing can cause major changes in your physical swing—and in where the ball goes.

For example, a single negative thought such as "Stay out of the bunker" or "Clear the water" can turn a good shot into a bad one. It's no accident that the best golfers are disciplined thinkers.

Tennis is the same as golf in respect to a single negative thought's power to spoil what otherwise would have been a good shot. The toughest competitors are the most disciplined thinkers, who follow a precise sequence of thinking and imaging during between-point time.

Getting tough *mentally* simply means learning when, how, and what to think and visualize to get the desired effect emotionally. Being tough *mentally* means that you have acquired skills in thinking, believing, and visualizing that enable you to:

- Readily access empowering emotions
- Quickly change from a negative emotional state to a positive one
- Cope emotionally with mistakes and failures
- Trigger an Ideal Performance State at will
- Cope with crisis and adversity

Mental toughness means that under pressure you can continue to think constructively, nondefensively, positively, and realistically with calmness and clarity.

STRATEGIES FOR LEARNING TOUGH THINKING

Getting tougher mentally calls for exercising your mind for the same reasons that toughening your body calls for exercising your muscles. Considering the vital part that mental agility plays in career success, it appears that surprisingly few people work specifically at increasing it. Instead, most simply seek to acquire knowledge and skills.

Abraham Lincoln saw the value of training his mind early in life, and forced himself to gain a complete understanding of Euclid's geometry. He knew the geometry would never be relevant to his life, but he mastered the subject anyway, purely for the mental training it gave him.

Find challenging subjects and activities, and spend a few hours each week studying them. Look for things that exercise your mind. Learn and play chess and other mentally challenging games, learn and use memorizing systems (a lot of good books have been published on this subject), study astronomy and math, do crossword puzzles, increase your vocabulary by looking up every unfamiliar word you encounter, learn a foreign language, master a new computer program. Today's world is full of exciting knowledge, new and old, that will exercise your brain.

All those activities provide opportunities for mental toughening. In the context of the Toughness Training for Life model, the following points are vital.

1. START ACKNOWLEDGING THAT WHAT YOU THINK HAS A SIGNIFICANT IMPACT ON HOW YOU FEEL

The connection between thought and emotion is real and direct. Thoughts don't merely float in your mind as so many people assume; they are electrochemical events even before they trigger emotions. And thoughts often trigger emotions instantly, by swiftly causing more chemical events to take place within the body.

Put a meter that records changes in skin moisture on almost anyone's finger and then show him or her a card with SPIDER printed on it. The meter indicator will instantly record a reaction. This happens even with people who profess no special fear of spiders and deny thinking about them much.

This means that if you start thinking about spiders, your body will react by secreting fear chemicals that match the level of your fear of spiders and your perception of the immediate threat of en- countering a big, ugly, hairy, poisonous spider that runs fast and can probably jump two feet. Just seeing spiders mentioned here probably raised your tension level so slightly that it could only be detected by a sensitive instrument. However, if you're either very good at visualizing or are uncommonly afraid of spiders, you may have felt symptoms of fear and increased tension, the demonstra- tion of which is the purpose of this paragraph.

Start thinking about a tragic event from your past and an emo- tion will immediately surface—sadness, anger, or whatever you really feel about that event. It may seem cold-blooded to "use" a per- sonal tragedy in any way, but this device from method acting is highly effective on occasions when it's important not to appear to feel jolly. Select a personal tragedy for this purpose that isn't too painful, one that won't make you feel guilty—unless that happens to be the way you want to look at a given moment.

To get positive emotions flowing—and to make it easier to put on your happy face when you need to but don't feel like it—think of fun times; recall the face of a loved one; recollect one of your stunning successes; remember a crack-up, belly-thumping joke; re- call a hilarious situation.

KEY POINT:

YOU CAN START YOUR BODY CHEMISTRY MOVING

IN WHATEVER DIRECTION YOU CHOOSE BY

DIRECTING YOUR THOUGHTS THAT WAY. EQUALLY

IMPORTANT, THE MORE YOU PRACTICE THIS

SKILL, THE BETTER YOU BECOME AT IT.

Negative thinking produces negative emotion, and negative emo- tion leads to negative thinking. It works both ways. It also works in the positive direction, where it will do you the most good. Positive thinking produces positive emotion, and positive emotion leads to positive thinking.

KEY POINT:

WHILE YOU CAN'T DIRECTLY CONTROL YOUR

FEELINGS, YOU CAN CONTROL YOUR THOUGHTS.

CONTROL THE DIRECTION AND CONTENT OF YOUR

THOUGHTS, AND YOU WILL EXERT CONSIDERABLE

CONTROL OVER HOW YOU FEEL.

2. TAKE FULL RESPONSIBILITY FOR WHAT AND HOW YOU THINK

Negative thoughts may intrude at any time and are certainly more prevalent during stressful periods. This means that during times of special stress you should be very conscious of the damaging power of negative thoughts.

While we may not always be able to prevent negative thoughts from appearing, we can choose not to entertain them. As soon as you realize you've let one sneak into your mind, you have two choices:

- You can dwell on the negative thought, hang on to it, twist it around in your mind and replay it over and over, and let it do every bit of damage it can.
- You can recast the negative thought in a positive light—or throw it out entirely and replace it with a wholly different but encouraging positive thought.

The quicker you get rid of a negative thought, the sooner you can get back to thinking the right stuff—something that will help you achieve your goal of the moment. Negative thinking never helped anyone do that.

Thinking the right stuff simply means entertaining the thoughts that will get you feeling empowered so you can solve the problem you face at that moment.

But you must start taking more responsibility for what you're thinking about and how you're thinking about it; otherwise, the right stuff will never get a chance to switch your emotional setting from negative to positive. In many situations, it has the same effect that taking your foot off the brake has when you step on the gas to move forward.

─────────────── **3.** START THINKING MORE FLEXIBLY ───────────────

Rigid thinking leads to rigid emotional responses. Rigid responses drive people to take inflexible actions that usually aren't in their best interests. Rigid thinking often hardens categories of emotional ruminations that often pass for thought, a hardening process that can seriously compromise your emotional flexibility.

For example:

"I'm always negative at work because I hate my boss. He's a total jerk." That's a thought only in the sense that it can occupy one's mind and fire up a negative emotion.

More flexible thinking: "I'm struggling to be positive at work because my boss and I are not connecting emotionally. He gets me feeling defensive and inferior. Since I can control my actions, attitudes, and thoughts but not his, what can I change that will improve the situation?"

Another example:

"I'm always unhappy at work because I hate my job."

More flexible thinking: "I'm having trouble being positive on the job because I find much of the work unfulfilling. What options can I open with my most innovative thinking that will lead to a promotion, a transfer, or the elimination of the least interesting parts of my job?"

Inflexible Thinking

Inflexible thinking is *nontough* thinking. Here are some habits of thinking or talking that hurt us emotionally:

- To say or think you *hate* something, someone, or some group of people. Examples: "I hate to travel." "I hate traffic." "I hate big cities." "I hate [whatever] food."
- To say or think you *can't* do something. Examples: "I can't

change." "I can't stand it." "I can't remember names (faces)." "I can't make myself heard."

- To say or think *never.* Examples: "I never get any breaks." "I'll never make it." "I'll never remember." "I'll never be able to do that." "I'll never be able to learn that."

How to Break the Inflexible Thinking Habit

If, like many of us, you regularly make things harder for yourself with some of those common nontough ways of inflexible thinking, how can you break the habit? The first step is to become aware of when and how you indulge yourself in rigid reactions.

Use the following list as a guide to spotting where you do your inflexible thinking, and what it consists of. Once you know what your inflexible habits are, you can start replacing them with flexible thinking that can help you.

COMMON *NONTOUGH* WAYS OF THINKING OR TALKING THAT HURT ME EMO-TIONALLY

1. During work_____
2. During sport activities _____
3. Under pressure _____
4. Following mistakes_____
5. During crisis _____
6. In general_____
7. While driving_____

Tough Thoughts

- I will put myself on the line every day.
- I will not surrender.
- I will not turn against myself during tough times.
- I will come totally prepared to compete every day.
- When it's tough, I will stay in control with humor.
- I will not show weakness on the outside.
- The crazier it gets, the more I will love it.
- I love competing more than winning.

─────────────── **4.** START THINKING MORE RESPONSIVELY ───────────────

It takes some mental effort, some commitment, but your efforts in this direction will quickly be well rewarded.

- Become very responsive mentally to psychological pain, that is, to negative feelings of any kind. If you feel hungry, tired, angry, frustrated, or any of the other litany of downers, figure out why and commit to doing something about it at your first opportunity. Then switch to positive thinking.
- Develop a keen mental awareness of negative emotional states such as depression, assumption of defeat, helplessness, and the like. Don't just accept them and muddle through; investigate why you feel that way, devise a solution, and put it into effect.
- Be very responsive mentally to the ringing phone of negative feelings. Your natural state is positive. When you're not feeling positive, there's a reason—pick up the phone and find out why.
- Imagine that you have a mental scanner that's always monitoring your emotional gauges. If you visualize this intensely, it will start working automatically, calling to your attention each time you stray into a negative emotional state. Remember, until you realize you've allowed yourself to slip into a negative mental state, you can't do anything about it, so an early-warning system is a mental must. Then at the first sign of negative thinking or emotion it will get your attention and you will mentally respond.

─────────────── **5.** START THINKING MORE ENERGETICALLY ───────────────

To get more positive emotion flowing, start talking and thinking more energetically. Here are some ways you can accomplish this vital mental toughening step:

- Think *fun,* and more positive energy will start flowing immediately.
- Think or say, "I love it," "Yes," and "Is this great or what?"

EXAMPLE: THE WORST TRAFFIC JAM IMAGINABLE
As enthusiastically as possible say, "Is this great traffic or what!" and then smile.

If there's nothing you can do to get out of the jam, isn't it point-less to work yourself into a highly negative emotional state? Instead, choose to be positive. Listen to an informational or inspirational tape on your tape deck. Mentally review your list of things to do. Think happy thoughts instead of angry thoughts. It's your choice. The point is, it's a habit of mind.

Instead of pounding your system with cortisol arousal—the old fight-or-flight response that worked great when primitive man saw a lion but won't do a thing for you in a traffic jam—practice willing yourself to be positive. It's a terrific opportunity to do that. Never let such an opportunity pass by without using it to intensify your mood-switching skills.

EXAMPLE: A DIFFICULT SALES CALL

As enthusiastically as possible, think and say, "I'm going to have some fun on this one. No hangdog look for me." Attitudes are contagious, and never more so than in a sales interview. Preparation and confidence are your most powerful weapons. Even if it was impossible for you to prepare as thoroughly as you'd like, you can still be confident.

EXAMPLE: A LONG, STRESSFUL DAY

You can let it beat you down, or you can beat the day down. Think and say, "Come on, there's got to be some fun in here somewhere." And then find it. Laughing under pressure is a learnable—and immensely valuable—mental toughening skill.

6. START THINKING MORE RESILIENTLY

Instead of letting negative feelings overwhelm you, think:
"I can get through this."
"This too will pass."
"I can handle this."
"I've been through worse things than this."
"Handling this is no sweat for a tough guy like me."
"This is not too much for me."
"I bounce back quickly."
"I'll be back."
"Tough times don't last but tough people do—and I'm tough."

————————— **7.** **START THINKING MORE HUMOROUSLY** —————————

It's a habit that can be acquired and used to displace the habit of thinking sourly or of always looking on the bad side of things. Here are some ways:

- Think nutty, goofy, silly, funny, off-the-wall thoughts. Never let yourself feel guilty about letting your mind run in these directions. It's the greatest therapy known to man.
- Think about things that break you up from the inside—things that make you start jiggling internally with laughter. Collect such things, treasure them, intensify them with repetition.

KEY POINT:

IN ALMOST EVERY SITUATION, BEING ABLE

TO LAUGH PUTS YOU IN EMOTIONAL CONTROL.

- The best and healthiest form of laughter is self-directed. People don't mind if you laugh at yourself—in fact, they'll usually happily join in. But laughing at them can leave scars that will last for years.
- The best humor is good-natured. It's directed at situations, not people.
- Avoid sarcasm. It's easy to fall into the habit of being sarcastic, especially to people who are unwilling, unable, or afraid to respond in kind. Sarcasm cuts like a knife, and can make serious enemies—a result that far outweighs the momentary pleasure of getting off a zinger.
- Take humor seriously. Skill with humor is an immensely valuable attribute. Miss no opportunity to improve your ability to use humor to smooth your way through life.

8. BE MORE DISCIPLINED IN THE WAY YOU REVIEW
YOUR MISTAKES AND FAILURES

There is only one excusable reason for reviewing mistakes and failures: to extract lessons from those experiences so you'll be less likely to repeat them. Reviewing mistakes and failures simply to punish yourself—engaging in pointless rehashes of things past and unchangeable—is one of the worst negative-thinking habits you can fall into.

- Sure, if it's possible, figure out why it happened. Ask yourself: "What could or should I have done differently?"
"What can I learn from this?"
"What can I take away from this that will help me in the future?"
- Treat it like a mission you've flown—debrief yourself and then make the conscious decision to *let it go!*
"It's over. I'm letting it go."
"It's history. I'm leaving the past behind."
"It's time to move on."
"It's okay. I can handle it. Now I'm moving forward again."

9. BE MORE DISCIPLINED IN THE WAY YOU THINK
ABOUT CRISIS AND ADVERSITY

Start by digging for a way to attribute some positive meaning to the crisis. Just adopting the determination to find positive meaning will help. Then move on to concede that you have to change how you do some things, live differently, accept some changes in your lifestyle or working methods. When you're faced with adversity, the longer you remain in denial, refusing the necessity of accepting changes, the longer you will remain in a negative, weakened state.

10. ASK YOURSELF QUESTIONS WHEN FACING
ADVERSITY OR CRISIS

"How can I use this event to grow and become stronger?"
"Is there a higher reason for this?"
"Can something good come of it?"
"Could this be a test for me?"

"Can this crisis get me back in touch with my real values?"
"What can I learn from this?"

---
11. THINK AND SAY WHAT YOU WANT TO FEEL
DURING THE CRISIS

You want to feel empowered, able to perform at your highest level.
This means that you need to be very positive in your thinking, because negative thoughts create negative feelings that will certainly
drag you further down. These methods will turn your thinking into
the positive state that will help you survive your crisis, and go on
to future success:

- Think and talk to yourself like a coach: "You can handle this."
  "Be strong." "Hang in there." "You can make it."
- Take a big picture view. In the total scheme of things, how bad
  is it? Tell yourself: "We still have each other." "We still have our
  health." "There's always next year." "Now we know more."

---
12. GET BACK TO BASICS DURING TOUGH TIMES

If you need to make adjustments, make them promptly and without
looking back. In everybody's life are a lot of nonvital activities and
expenditures that can be put aside, if only temporarily.

- Use the crisis to reestablish your *real* priorities in life.
- Bring your *core* values and beliefs to life. Ask yourself: "What is
  really important here?"
- Take action according to your *core* values. Be decisive and clear-
  thinking in a crisis, building from your core beliefs:

Love	Honesty
Caring	Sincerity
Family	Support
Integrity	Health

Reviewing your core beliefs is a powerful way of helping yourself cope with crisis and adversity. It helps to write them down:

MY CORE BELIEFS ARE:

1. _____

2. _____

3. _____

4. _____

5. _____

—————————— **13. USE POSITIVE VISUALIZATION TO CHANGE** ——————————
—————————— **NEGATIVE EMOTIONAL STATES TO POSITIVE ONES** ——————————

- A vivid mental picture is worth a thousand words. Images are
  much more powerful than words in stimulating emotion. Here's
  a way to practice the kind of vivid visualization that's effective in
  altering your emotional state. Our examples are for negative visualization, because those images are more universal and the
  concept can be more easily grasped.

  However, you don't need to practice negative visualization;
  the chances are you can already do that far more effectively
  than is really helpful.
- Do your visualization practice with warm and happy or deeply
  pleasurable images taken from your private life.

VIVID VISUALIZATION EXAMPLE:
Picture yourself on a camping trip. A snake has crawled into your
sleeping bag. See exactly what it looks like. Feel its cold, slimy
body as it moves across your chest.

When you visualize something like that, fear is instantly
triggered—more powerfully than by simply thinking about it with
words instead of with images and feelings.

- When you can't immediately fulfill a strong need, you continue
  to experience a lot of negative emotion because the need remains unfulfilled (the phone keeps on ringing loudly). Handle
  this by visualizing in detail exactly how you intend to meet the
  need. See and feel it happen in your imagination.
- Visualize strongly enough to feel the relief and pleasure you'll
  experience when your need is met. For example, how much fun
  you'll have when the weekend comes; how good you'll feel when

you finally have that talk with your boss; how good you'll feel when the speech you're so worried about is finally over; how good you'll feel when you're finally snuggled down in bed ready to sleep.

- Visualizing the need being positively fulfilled will bring temporary relief (the phone will stop ringing for a while), which will allow you to return to a positive emotional state.

KEY POINT:

YOUR CENTRAL NERVOUS SYSTEM CAN'T

TELL THE DIFFERENCE BETWEEN SOMETHING

VIVIDLY IMAGINED AND SOMETHING THAT

ACTUALLY HAPPENED.

- That key point means that your central nervous system can be fooled into believing the need has been met. This buys a little more time to function without the cloud of negative emotion hanging over you. But you must still legitimately meet the unfulfilled need as soon as possible or the painful ringing will start again.
- Give meaning to your emotional pain and give yourself temporary permission not to experience it. To help you do that, answer these questions:
  - What am I feeling right now?
  - If I'm feeling negative, why? What is the unfulfilled need?
- Keep in mind that psychological pain always serves a purpose. With practice, you'll start getting much better at understanding the meaning and significance of your negative emotional state. Once you commit to fulfilling the need as soon as possible and give yourself temporary permission to no longer experience the pain, you may have to insist that the phone no longer be allowed to ring for a designated period of time.

JUST FOR TODAY

JUST FOR TODAY
I will become challenged when problems come my way. Today I will be a great problem solver.

JUST FOR TODAY
I will love the battle. I can create my own state of enjoyment. I will accept the hand that is dealt to me. No complaining!

JUST FOR TODAY
I will exercise, eat, and train right. Self-discipline will bring the confidence I search for.

JUST FOR TODAY
I will take charge of how I feel. I will not be at the mercy of my emotions.

JUST FOR TODAY
I will set aside time to relax and simply let go. Recovery is an essential part of my training.

JUST FOR TODAY
I will have a plan to follow. The plan will keep me focused and organized.

JUST FOR TODAY
I will stop saying, "If I had time." If I want time, I will take it.

JUST FOR TODAY
I will find humor in my mistakes. When I can smile inside, I am in control.

JUST FOR TODAY
I will do things the best I can. I will be satisfied with what I have done.

JUST FOR TODAY

I will do the ordinary things in my training extraordinarily well. It's the little things that make the difference.

JUST FOR TODAY

I choose to believe that I can make the difference and that I am in control of my world.

The choice is mine.

11

TOUGHENING

THE IMMUNE

SYSTEM

The battle rages without pause. Hordes of enemy invaders relentlessly probe for any weakness on perimeter walls that will let them break through and overrun the defenders. Although the invaders are crafty and persistent, they face one of the most ingenious defense systems imaginable. Biological warfare units, alert Pac-Man-like sentinels, chemical killing agents, scanners, specialized weapons of all kinds, and even highly efficient killing squads leap into the fray at a moment's notice.

No, this is not science fiction, *Star Wars* or a newly released sequel to the movie thriller *Alien*. This is real. And the fighting isn't raging in some faraway place like Iraq or Croatia. It's the daily reality in your own body, where your immune system fights desperately to keep you alive.

Simply put, our immune system rivals the greatest marvels in all life. Probing the vast frontiers of the human immune response can easily leave one awestruck at its genius, power, and scope.

The tragic AIDS epidemic has focused worldwide research on

the immune system. The AIDS virus attacks one of the most critical units of immune defense, the helper T cell, and by so doing eventually undermines the entire system.

In a most insidious fashion, the AIDS virus enters the body and conceals itself within a helper T cell. Before the unsuspecting T cell can mount an attack, the AIDS virus disables it. AIDS provides dramatic evidence of what happens when the immune system is weakened.

LINKING EMOTIONS WITH THE IMMUNE RESPONSE

In the second century, the Greek physician Galen noted that disease is a consequence of psychic imbalance. That belief prevailed in the practice of medicine for more than a millennium. With the advent of modern medical science, however, the contention that mental and emotional states influence the body's disease-fighting capacity was rejected.

Only in the past 20 years has the connection between psychological factors and immune function been seriously reexplored. Leading the search is the new field of psychoneuroimmunology (PNI). PNI researchers focus principally on how the brain and the body's immune system interact.

A VITAL LINK BETWEEN BRAIN AND BODY

A rich network of blood vessels links the hypothalamus (the brain's autonomic center) to the pituitary (the body's master gland). Discovering this network has helped researchers understand how thoughts and emotions affect the immune system.

For years, immunologists have suspected that the hormones of stress directly influence the immune response. The understanding that thoughts and emotions are biochemical events—and that as such they can send messages from brain cells to immune cells—also helped researchers move forward.

Several studies in recent years have shown positive links between emotional factors and immune response. Increased incidence of cancer has been associated with patients described as being repressed, sad, bland, helpless, stoic, unassertive, eager to please, passive, fearful, or hopeless.

Loneliness, psychological distress, depression, pressure to perform, and low social support have also been shown to correlate with immune suppression, as well as with certain types of cancers, and with poorer disease prognosis.

Fighting spirit, the will to live, emotional expressiveness, and optimism have been linked to immune enhancement and health. The release of negative emotion through verbal or written expression has also been linked to increased immune effectiveness.

THE IMMUNE SYSTEM TALKS BACK

Many PNI researchers now believe that communication between the brain and the immune system works both ways. The brain talks to the immune system using an automatic by-product of conscious thought and emotion, and the immune system talks back. According to PNI researcher Nicholas Hall, the immune system responds much as a sensory organ does. It is capable of sending and receiving messages throughout the body regarding invading viruses and bacteria.

Hall contends that immune cells not only attack the invading organisms but also stimulate changes throughout the body to help fight the intruders. These changes affect such things as temperature, hormone release, and sleep.

Evidence that communication exists between brain and immune system comes from many directions. The lymph nodes are one of the immune system's principal groups of organs. Filled with nerve fibers that act like telephone trunk lines, the lymph nodes send and receive messages to and from the entire body. Special chemicals called neurotransmitters attach themselves to immune cells and influence their disease-fighting potential.

Researchers at Ohio State University College of Medicine studied the immune systems of married women. They found that marital happiness, decreased depression, and reduced loneliness are associated with healthier immune systems.

Arthur Stone and his colleagues at New York State University studied the moods and immune response of 30 dental students. They found that bad moods and relatively low antibody production occurred on the same days. Good moods were associated with a bolstered antibody immune response.

Researchers at New Mexico University's School of Medicine studied 256 healthy elderly people. They found that a strong interpersonal support system significantly improved immune function.

THE LANGUAGE OF EMOTION

An important part of the brain's messages to the immune cells are clearly emotional. With equal clarity we know that the messages are mainly carried by hormonal messengers.

Neuroresearcher Candace Pert contends that brain cells produce small proteinlike chemicals called neuropeptides to provide the chemical basis of emotion. Neuropeptides have powerful mood-stimulating effects. High concentrations of them are found in the limbic system of the brain, thought to be the control center of emotion.

Endorphins are examples of neuropeptides. When immune cells (lymphocytes) encounter bacteria or viruses, they send chemical messages to the brain via the blood. These messages speed up or slow down the activity of the immune system. In all probability, the chemical messages of the emotions are communicated in the same way. Research has already confirmed that endorphins stimulate immune cells through such a message network.

One of the ways the brain influences the immune system's activities is through pituitary-adrenal arousal; the response we learned earlier in Chapter 6 is stimulated during times of distress and negative emotion. At those times, stress hormones such as cortisol and ACTH are released.

Increased susceptibility to disease and reduced immune responsiveness have been linked to lengthy episodes during which higher than normal levels of those hormones remained in the blood. Intense and persistent periods of negative emotion such as fear, helplessness, depression, and grieving have been shown to suppress normal immune functions.

HOW THE IMMUNE SYSTEM LEARNS OF POSITIVE EMOTION

Researchers now believe that positive emotional states can be transmitted to the immune system in either or both of two ways: (1) indirectly through hormone release, (2) directly through the complex neural pathways of the autonomic nervous structure, pathways that extend to nearly all components of the immune system.

KEY POINT:

OUR THOUGHTS AND FEELINGS AFFECT OUR BODY'S

DISEASE-FIGHTING POTENTIAL TO AN IMPORTANT DEGREE.

USING THE COMMUNICATION CHANNELS OF EMOTION

The communication channels are there, waiting to be used to the fullest extent possible. Many of us already use those channels naturally, usually only to a limited degree.

Mostly we do it as chance dictates. Few understand how to use those precious channels between mind and body, between our thoughts/feelings and our health, as deliberately, regularly, and as intensely as we easily could. This is unfortunate.

Research has confirmed that we can strengthen the immune system with laughter, happiness, confidence, and the whole range of positive emotions. To achieve the highest level of health that we're capable of attaining, we need to establish positive thoughts and feelings as our normal attitude.

As we toughen mentally and emotionally, as we gain more control over positive and negative arousal cycles, we simultaneously gain greater control over our immune response.

KEY POINT:

OUR ABILITY TO FIGHT OFF DISEASE LARGELY PARALLELS

OUR ABILITY TO CONTROL OUR THOUGHTS AND EMOTIONS.

—— HOW STRESS STRENGTHENS AND WEAKENS YOUR IMMUNE SYSTEM ——

Just as we learned that a healthy muscle is flexible, responsive, strong, and resilient, so also is your body's immune system. A healthy, toughened immune system is flexible, responsive, and strong when challenged by an invader, and it recovers quickly after winning each of its battles.

And just as we have learned that stress is vital for the healthy development and functioning of muscles, the same principle applies to our immune apparatus. A good example is the immune system's thymus gland.

The thymus gland, essentially a proving ground for immature immune cells, must be exposed to a certain level of stress for healthy development to occur. That is, the thymus must have the opportunity to fight off invading bacteria or it won't develop. When animals are experimentally raised in a germ-free environment from birth, their thymus glands are severely underdeveloped compared to those of animals raised in normal conditions. As a result, the overly protected animals live only a short time outside their original germ-free environment before disease overwhelms their stunted immune systems.

—————— HOW STRESS AND THE IMMUNE SYSTEM ARE RELATED ——————

Comprehending the interrelationship of stress and the immune system requires an understanding of the arousal sequence of stress. Both psychological and physical stress stimulate the limbic system that lies deep within the brain. Emotional messages of threat, fun, fear, challenge, and so on are relayed directly through neural pathways (nerves) or indirectly via chemical messengers.

The messages are eventually received by the hypothalamus, which serves as a bridge between the brain and the endocrine system. Messages of distress such as anger, fear, and depression then travel two or three centimeters to stimulate the pituitary gland.

After receiving the distress call, the pituitary gland magnifies it by secreting a hormone called ACTH (adrenocorticotropic hormone). ACTH stimulates the outer layer of the adrenal gland.

The immune response can become jeopardized at this point. Corticosteroids released by the adrenal gland clearly serve to suppress the immune system's response capability. Cortisol is one of the principal corticosteroid hormones responsible for the suppression. It should be noted, however, that minimal levels of cortisol are necessary for immune activation.

Why do signals of distress and negative emotion cause immune suppression?

It's a curious enigma. What possible reason could nature have for linking negative stress (physical or psychological pain) with the immune system? Several plausible explanations have been offered by immunologists, but the most widely accepted one points to energy preservation. Temporarily diverting energy away from the internal immune wars constantly raging on many fronts within the body permits more energy to be summoned to face the perceived threat from outside. The greater the perceived threat and the attendant negative emotion, the greater the degree of immune suppression.

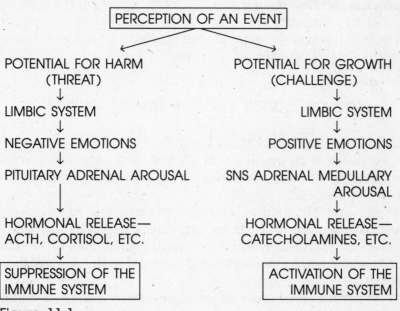

Figure 11.1

Suspending various components of the immune system *temporarily* to conserve energy is not really a problem. Again the culprit is linear negative stress for extended periods of time without relief. For instance, intense grieving from the loss of a loved one without breaks can have tragic immune consequences. Grieving in cycles, however, can usually be managed.

In addition to linearity, the component of helplessness also appears to block or suppress immune response. Several researchers have discovered that simply the perception of control can prevent adverse immune reactions. Animal research also supports these findings.

The immune systems of mice were not adversely affected when the mice were stressed with electric shock provided they were able to escape or in some way control the shock. Inability to control a stressor and inability to achieve periodic relief from a stressor, as in the case of overcrowding and isolation, invariably had debilitating effects on the immune systems of mice.

From all the available evidence, toughening the immune system, like toughening muscles, occurs in response to intermittent exposure to stress. Similarly, weakening occurs in response to insufficient stress, inadequate recovery, or excessive stress—especially excessive negative stress. The same toughening principles that apply to muscles and emotions apply to the immune system. That is an exciting discovery.

PHYSICAL STRESS AND THE IMMUNE RESPONSE

In the early 1900s, researchers began linking physical exercise with susceptibility to certain illnesses. Their studies suggested a correlation between physical stress and lowered immune system effectiveness.

For example, in 1918, Cowles discovered a strong connection between pneumonia and other respiratory infections and intense prolonged exercise. Acute poliomyelitis was found to be much more severe when intense exercise occurred at the onset of the infection.

Overtraining in sport as well as excessive competitive stress have been linked to increased susceptibility to infectious mononucleosis and upper respiratory illnesses of all kinds. Chronic fatigue and increased incidence of colds and flu have also been linked to overtraining in sport.

Research over the past four decades indicates that athletes who train intensely for long periods of time without adequate rest and those who expose themselves to massive doses of exercise stress (such as an ultramarathon) are at greatest risk of an impaired immune response.

In 1983, researchers Peters and Bateman studied 140 runners before and after an ultramarathon. Compared with a matched control group, runners had over twice as many upper respiratory infections following the race as the control group. Of particular interest was the finding that as race times decreased, the incidence of illness increased; this suggests a connection between the physical stress response and the immune response.

A similar study was conducted in 1990 of participants in the Los Angeles Marathon. Results showed that the marathon runners were five times more likely to become ill following the race than trained runners who did not enter the race.

LABORATORY RATS AND EXERCISE

For obvious ethical reasons, it is not possible for researchers to design controlled studies in which subjects are exposed to excessive doses of physical stress (overtraining) to study the link between exercise and the immune response. Based on controlled animal research studies, however, the following statements are supportable:

- Moderate exercise training prior to infection enhances resistance.
- Moderate to intense exercise at the time of infection, or following the infection, reduces resistance.
- Resistance to viral infection can be severely compromised by poorly timed episodes of intense and prolonged physical exercise.
- Prior exercise training can strengthen immune response against potential viral infection.

Of particular significance is the consensus by animal researchers that high levels of corticosteroids, most notably cortisol, are associated with suppression of the immune system.

──────────── GIVING YOUR IMMUNE SYSTEM A WORKOUT ────────────

The possibility that one might be able to use certain kinds of exercise to toughen the immune system is certainly exciting. The question is how.

How can the stress of exercise cause immune cells to become more flexible, responsive, strong, or resilient? Could it be that the hormones released during exercise actually *stress* immune cells into moving or oscillating?

The answer is yes, they do.

Researchers have found that the numbers of a particular type of immune cell called a leukocyte increase during exercise as much as four times over resting levels. The rate of increase depends on the duration and intensity of the exercise and the fitness level of the exerciser.

Researchers also confirmed that the count of another type of immune cell, the lymphocyte, significantly increases both during and immediately following exercise. However, lymphocyte numbers *decrease* below resting levels following long-distance marathon-type running—a finding of particular importance. As an example, researchers Nieman and Berk found that the lymphocyte count was 20 percent lower than resting levels following a three-hour run.

Highly significant also was the discovery that NK cells, meaning Natural Killer cells, increased in number as much as 300 percent during and following exercise. NK activity returned to normal within one hour of the exercise when the exercise duration was 30 minutes or less. In cases of prolonged exercise, however, NK numbers actually *decreased,* a condition lasting between one and six hours. This suggests that the immune stress was excessive. The findings held constant for all ages including those over the age of 65.

Finally, the numbers of another immune cell called the B cell dramatically increased during exercise and quickly returned to normal following moderate exercise stress.

The collective evidence strongly supports the notion that the immune system gets a workout from exercise in much the same way the muscular and cardiovascular systems do. A moderate dose of physical stress gets the immune chemistry moving, and that movement can lead to increased immune toughness.

────────── **KEY TIPS FOR STRENGTHENING YOUR IMMUNE SYSTEM** ──────────

Here are some important understandings about exercise that can help you strengthen your immune system:

- Creating numerous low to moderate waves of physical stress intermittently throughout the day will enhance the immune function if the exercise is balanced by proper recovery.
- Positive arousal in the form of short-term catecholamine release during exercise can strengthen the immune response.
- Prolonged catecholamine release because of excessive physical exercise leads to catecholamine depletion. This weakens the immune response.
- Toughening a deficient immune system can be accomplished by applying controlled doses of physical stress in the same way we toughen our muscles and emotions.
- The increases in catecholamine levels that accompany exercise are largely responsible for the increased number of immune cells circulating in the blood.
- Muscle contraction during exercise also contracts lymphatic tissue, resulting in greater circulation and movement of immune cells throughout the body.

As we learned in Chapter 6 from Richard Dienstbier's toughening model, intermittent doses of physical stress lead to three things:

1. *Lower resting levels of catecholamines.* This seems to allow normal immune activity to continue under conditions of minimal stress.
2. *Greater resistance to catecholamine depletion.* Immune function deteriorates as the catecholamines become depleted.
3. *Suppressed adrenal-cortical responses* (negative arousal). The release of immune-suppressing agents associated with negative arousal, such as cortisol, is suppressed.

MORE EVIDENCE THAT EXERCISE
STRENGTHENS IMMUNITY

Several longitudinal studies covering spans of 10 to 20 years have reported significantly fewer cancers in men and women who remain physically active. In a study published in 1989, researchers Albanes, Blair, and Taylor found that inactive men had an 80 percent greater risk of cancer than active men. In a related study, Barbash and his colleagues found the risk of colon cancer was nearly two times greater in occupational groups that remained largely inactive than in more physically active groups.

In 1985, a study of over 5,000 college alumni revealed that breast and reproductive system cancer was consistently more prevalent among nonathletes. Former athletes have been shown to exercise more than nonathletes. Lower rates of lung, thyroid, and digestive cancer have also been reported for active compared to inactive groups.

For over forty years, research with animals has shown positive relationships between the inhibition of experimentally induced tumors and exercise. The collective evidence strongly supports the contention that moderate exercise inhibits the growth of animal tumors.

Best results were obtained when exercise routines began several weeks before the tumor was implanted and were continued as long as tumor growth was to be inhibited. The inhibitory effects of the physical exercise continued only as long as the exercise did.

DRUGS AND IMMUNITY

KEY POINT:

ONE OF THE GREATEST THREATS TO THE IMMUNE

SYSTEM IS THE RECREATIONAL USE OF DRUGS.

Increasing evidence links immune suppression with the use of hypodermic needles to self-administer such drugs as cocaine and morphine. Even nonintravenous use of such drugs as marijuana, amphetamines, Quaaludes, LSD, cocaine, and PCP have been shown to have immune-suppressive side effects. The link between AIDS and drug abuse continues to grow. Estimates are that as many as 50 to 75 percent of AIDS patients in the United States had compromised immune systems because of some form of drug abuse before infection with AIDS.

THE POWER OF BELIEF

In 1950, the drug Krebiozen received national publicity as a sensational wonder cure for cancer. The American Medical Association and the Food and Drug Administration began a thorough testing program to study the scientific validity of the drug.

Dr. Bruno Klopfer was one of many physicians who became involved with testing Krebiozen. He did so because one of his patients, a man with an advanced lymphosarcoma malignancy, read about the amazing power of Krebiozen and pleaded with Dr. Klopfer to get involved in the study. The patient had large tumor masses throughout his body and was in extremely poor physical condition.

Following administration of the drug, the patient made a rapid and startling recovery. His tumors shrank dramatically and within a short time he resumed a completely normal life. However, when he read reports from the AMA and FDA that Krebiozen had proved to be ineffective against cancer, the man took a sudden turn for the worse.

Realizing his patient was deteriorating fast, Dr. Klopfer told him he had obtained a super-strength form of Krebiozen that produced far superior results. Following administration of the "new" drug—in reality only sterile water—the patient again showed remarkable recovery. The tumor masses seemed to melt away, Klopfer reported.

The patient remained symptom-free for over two months until he again read further reports about the failure of Krebiozen to "cure" cancer. Within a few days of hearing that news, the patient died.

The sudden and dramatic improvement of Dr. Klopfer's patient was the result of what science calls the "placebo effect." Every medical practitioner knows this sugar-pill phenomenon.

Placebos are often dramatically effective in treating diseases of all kinds. As cancer specialist Carl Simonton asserts, "The only active ingredient in the treatment appears to be the power of the belief, the positive expectations."

Researchers are painfully aware that without rigid and precise control procedures, the placebo effect can completely contaminate research findings with false positives. Worthless drugs, therapies, and health interventions of all kinds show statistical significance.

Countless examples of sudden dramatic reversal of disease from placebo cures have been documented throughout medical history. Practices that we now know have no medical basis whatsoever, such as bleeding, produced remarkable results. The only factor common to these bogus "cures" was the power of belief. Faith healing, healing miracles, and many examples of spontaneous remission of symptoms all seem to involve a strong, intense belief that the "cure" will work.

From the research perspective, the placebo effect is simply a maddening nuisance that complicates the task of finding truth. In the context of Toughness Training, however, the placebo effect is dramatic, undeniable evidence that a direct link exists between emotions and the immune system.

GREAT NEWS!

THE POWER OF THE PLACEBO IS LIVING PROOF OF BELIEF'S POWER.

OUR BELIEFS AND EMOTIONS ARE LARGELY CONTROLLABLE BY

CONTROLLING HOW WE THINK AND ACT.

THEREFORE WE CAN INVOKE THE PLACEBO EFFECT AT WILL, AND PUT

THE FULL POWER OF BELIEF TO WORK AT ACHIEVING ANY GOAL WE

CHOOSE.

This means that our immune system is within our reach. In addition to exercise, thinking tough and acting tough can actively toughen our immune system in important ways.

SOME ADDITIONAL IMMUNE INSIGHTS

1. FAULTY IMMUNE SYSTEMS MAY CAUSE EMOTIONAL PROBLEMS.

Because communication works both ways between the brain and the immune cells, researchers are exploring how the immune system's actions can impact emotional states. Some of the brain chemicals triggered by immune activity—such as neurotransmitters and neuropeptides—are associated with emotional states.

Nick Hall and others suspect that some psychiatric disorders may be the result of faulty immune responses. Since the release of such powerful hormones as cortisol and ACTH as well as a host of catecholamines can be stimulated both ways, the immune system's involvement in some behavioral and psychiatric disorders certainly seems plausible.

2. BY ITSELF, THE IMMUNE SYSTEM PRODUCES POWERFUL NEUROHORMONES.

Ed Blalock, an immunologist at the University of Alabama, was one of the first to discover that immune cells actually make endorphins, ACTH, and growth hormones. Blalock believes that the capacity to generate such a wide diversity of hormones enables the immune system to influence nearly every other system of the body.

3. VISUALIZATION MAY ENHANCE THE IMMUNE FUNCTION.

French researcher Gerard Renoux discovered that in mice, the left hemisphere of the brain activates the immune system and the right side suppresses it. Renoux theorizes that humans have a similar, yet far more complex configuration. His theory helps explain why visualization may play a positive role in fighting cancer.

Visualization and imaging mainly stimulate the right side of the brain—the side believed to be involved in immune suppression. Renoux speculates that visualization may distract the right hemisphere from suppression, thus allowing the immune response to function at higher than normal levels.

Some evidence also exists that the left hemisphere of the brain processes and integrates positive emotions and the right side negative ones. Visualization and positive imaging may also work to suppress negative arousal states associated with pituitary-adrenal stimulation. Suppression of cortisol and ACTH, as we learned earlier, enhances immune function.

SUMMARY

Conservative medical experts generally agree that as much as 75 percent of human illness is stress-related. Excessive, uncontrolled stress can ravage our immune systems, leaving our bodies vulnerable to attack.

When our health is seriously jeopardized, everything else suddenly pales in importance. Clearly, health is our most precious asset, but too often we fail to recognize that reality until the battle is nearly lost.

Actively toughening our immune system protects this supreme resource. We can and must accept more responsibility for our own health—the price for not doing so is simply too high.

Disease is the consequence of immune failure that is most often rooted in some form of stress/recovery imbalance. Excessive stress, insufficient stress, excessive recovery, and insufficient recovery are all potential culprits.

Toughening our immune systems means controlling cycles of stress and recovery in precisely the same ways that we have learned to toughen our muscles and cardiovascular systems. The basic formula for toughening our immune systems is simple. Here it is:

- Fulfill your basic needs for sleep, food, and water in the healthiest, most direct, and consistent ways possible. Solid nutrition is a must!
- Use regular, moderate exercise to actively strengthen your immune response. Eighty percent of your exercise intervals should be within your aerobic target range; 20 percent can be below or above your range. Only experienced exercisers who have no known risk factors should go above the 80 percent limit.
- Break up periods of linear stress—whether physical, emotional or mental—with regular periods of *trained recovery.*

TOUGHENED IMMUNE SYSTEM

Flexible, responsive,
strong, and resilient
under attack

Step 3

TOUGHEN MENTALLY

- Disciplined thinking and imaging under stress
- Strong beliefs and values
- Thinking "tough"

Step 2

TOUGHEN PHYSICALLY

- Physical challenge with exercise
- Looking "tough" under stress

Step 1

BUILD SOUND RECOVERY BASE

Good nutrition, sleep, rest

Figure 11.2   The Building Blocks of Immune Toughening

- Control the frequency and intensity of cycles of negative arousal because of the immune-suppressive effects of such hormones as cortisol and ACTH.
- Use the power of belief, positive visualization, and positive expectation to enhance immune response. Remember, the placebo effect is real!

PARAMOUNT POINT:

YOUR GOAL SHOULD BE TO DEVELOP A TOUGHENED

IMMUNE SYSTEM THAT WILL REMAIN FLEXIBLE,

RESPONSIVE, STRONG, AND RESILIENT AGAINST ALL ODDS.

THIS IS A *MUST*-WIN BATTLE.

12

PARENTING

TOUGH KIDS:

HOW IT'S DONE

Many parents shudder to think what the world will be like when their children reach maturity. Uncertainty, change, and stress are far more deeply woven into the fabric of today's life than was the case a generation ago. These ominous trends are so pervasive that one can only speculate about how tough people will have to be to find happiness and success in tomorrow's world.

Parents are becoming increasingly concerned that their children simply won't be tough enough to meet the challenges they will inevitably face as adults. The world is definitely going to get tougher—so must our children if they're to have any chance at all.

Sending nontough young adults forward to meet their futures will likely have tragic consequences. As parents, we must find better ways to accelerate the toughening process because the stakes are so high. The happiness, health, and productivity of each of our children are on the line.

The problem isn't only that the world is getting tougher. Many of today's kids would be ill prepared for the less tough worlds of yesteryear, let alone the future they will live or die in. The problem is a tremendous upsurge in kids who are woefully soft physically.

Until recently it was rare for children to suffer muscle degeneration from inactivity. Their perpetual motion was always the delight and despair of parents. Today, however, the temptations of TV watching, the advent of the latch-key generation, and the dangers of the streets have drastically reduced the physical activity of millions of children.

Thanks to several hours of TV watching a day combined with high-fat snacks, more and more children are overweight, a development that has ominous implications for the health of 21st-century Americans. Only a lucky few today enjoy a childhood of constant physical activity in the Huckleberry Finn tradition. Even fewer will in the future unless parents take strong measures.

The creation of overweight and underexercising adults often begins in early childhood and accelerates steadily as time passes. As a result, many of today's children won't have the physical ruggedness and energy that young people need to survive and prosper against the challenges of adulthood. Instead, they will reach adulthood and obesity at the same time.

Parents of today's children thus face a doubled challenge: the contemporary pull toward health-threatening physical softness, and certainty that tomorrow's world will be a tougher place to fight life's battles.

Here are some of the questions this chapter proposes to answer:

- Why are some kids tough and others not?
- Which parental practices weaken kids and which strengthen them?
- How can parents accelerate the toughening process so their kids will get the best possible preparation for the future?
- What specifically can parents do to develop flexibility, responsiveness, strength, and resiliency in their children?

13 WAYS TO RAISE TOUGHER KIDS

1. RESPOND TO YOUR CHILDREN'S BASIC PHYSIOLOGICAL RECOVERY
   NEEDS.

Parents who fail to meet their children's needs for food, sleep, rest, and stimulation virtually guarantee that the foundation for toughness won't be put in place. Basic needs that go unanswered in a child's early years perpetuate physiological and psychological disharmony and disorder that spawn chronic distrust and feelings of helplessness.

A world that is unresponsive to children's expressions of physical need undermines their sense of personal control. Anger, fear, and negative arousal become habitual daily realities. Unmet basic physiological needs are simply forms of overtraining that can lead to the failure of all recovery mechanisms.

2. RESPOND WARMLY AND DEPENDABLY TO YOUR CHILDREN'S BASIC
   EMOTIONAL RECOVERY NEEDS.

Needs for safety, security, love, and affection are among the most critical forms of recovery during early development. Affection and warmth in childhood are strong predictors of happiness and health in adulthood.

Loving is recovery. Love is the principal mechanism through which the child learns to balance psychological distress in the form of fear, insecurity, and emotional pain.

A classic study by Boston University's Carol Franz spanned a period of 36 years. Franz discovered that children from warm and affectionate families were consistently more motivated, happier, and more stable as adults than children from unaffectionate parents. Affection and warmth proved to be far more important than structure and discipline in producing strong, healthy adults.

In much the same way as unmet basic physiological needs, inadequate emotional recovery that stems from insufficient love and affection becomes *overtraining.* Cycles of emotional stress simply cannot be balanced without the recovery achieved from love and affection.

3. USE EXERCISE TO TOUGHEN YOUR CHILDREN.

The way to raise physically active kids is to be physically active yourself. It's never been more important. Many of today's kids are virtually motionless all day at school and continue to be motionless at home for hours on end in front of television sets. Seven hours of physical inactivity at school followed by six hours of TV constitute serious *physical undertraining*.

The cornerstones of toughness—flexibility, responsiveness, strength, and resiliency—are physically eroded by such a routine. All too often, weak physically means weak emotionally. Problems of low energy, overeating, and poor endurance are natural companions of poor fitness.

Ironically, our children are becoming less fit at a time in history when their toughness will be challenged more than ever before, both as children and as adults. Parents don't exercise and toughen physically, so neither do their children. Both tragically fail to utilize one of the most powerful accelerators of toughness that is available.

4. AVOID OVERTRAINING YOUR KIDS BY SAYING NO TOO OFTEN, AND UNDERTRAINING THEM BY NOT SAYING NO OFTEN ENOUGH.

To a child who wants something, *no* is stress and *yes* is recovery. All too often parents confuse *yes* with love and *no* with a lack of love, overlooking the fact that the real world is not a *yes* kind of place.

Too many yeses and not enough noes spoils children by overprotecting them. As a consequence, they are never adequately toughened for the ego-crunching noes of adult life.

Saying yes too often can weaken children by undertraining them; saying no too often can weaken children by overtraining them. Saying no becomes a particularly critical issue when it involves basic physical or emotional recovery needs. Toughening requires consistent yeses to basic needs and periodic, compassionate noes to nonessential ones.

5. DON'T USE FEAR AS YOUR MAIN WAY TO CONTROL AND MOTIVATE YOUR CHILDREN.

Fear works. Parents can get their kids to do amazing things by using or threatening physical or emotional pain. Physical punishment, rejection, and the withdrawal of love are indeed powerful weapons in a parent's arsenal.

However, parents who persistently use fear to control their children chronically stimulate negative arousal and, in so doing, undermine an essential component of toughness.

Fearful children become fearful adults. A child who is controlled by fear—fear of making mistakes, guilt, fear of failure, fear of rejection, fear of loving—will inevitably acquire nontough ways of thinking and acting.

6. AVOID OVERTRAINING YOUR CHILDREN WITH EXCESSIVE PRESSURE TO ACHIEVE.

High-achieving parents are especially prone to act counterproductively in this way. To prevent laziness and low motivation from blocking their children's achievement, parents become the driving force.

They constantly exert great pressure on their children to be number one, to excel at everything they do. Nothing but the best is acceptable.

This pressure for high achievement at everything creates a highly linear form of stress that allows few opportunities for full recovery. Because most people simply cannot be number one at everything they do, the feelings of failure, guilt, and inadequacy that were ingrained in childhood become everyday adult realities.

7. DON'T BE RIGID, INFLEXIBLE, AND ROUGH.

Some parents wrongly equate rigid and rough child-rearing practices with producing tough kids. Cold, rough, inflexible parenting produces cold, rigid, defensive children.

Parents who bend the rules occasionally are not necessarily weak. Flexible parenting often signals parental warmth, perspective, compassion, and openness.

Tough kids don't emerge from rough handling. Tough kids are those who have learned to get their basic physiological and psychological needs met in healthy ways. As a result, they can absorb emotional hits with flexibility and resiliency. Rough handling does not accelerate that process.

8. TEACH YOUR CHILDREN HOW TO INTERPRET AND RESPOND TO
   RECOVERY'S LANGUAGE.

Children need to begin to learn how to decode body talk as early
in their development as possible. Learning how to listen and interpret the language of recovery is a prerequisite for meeting one's
needs in a healthy, timely fashion.

Three fundamental sensitivities should begin to be acquired in
childhood:

- Understanding the message behind physical and psychological
  pain
- Understanding the meaning of negative emotion
- Understanding that a negative state of mind is not normal

Children need to know that feelings have a purpose and are to be
valued. They also need to know that the first step in being responsive to one's basic needs is listening. Only then can the real need
behind fatigue, sadness, anger, depression, or confusion be met.
Once learned, these are lifetime skills.

9. TEACH YOUR CHILDREN HOW TO SPIKE AND TROUGH THEIR CHEMISTRY
   IN HEALTHY WAYS.

If kids are not taught how to naturally spike periods of exciting
arousal and trough periods of deep relief in healthy ways, they are
enormously more likely to learn unhealthy ways on their own. The
point is that, like it or not, kids will figure out some way to oscillate.

Drugs, sex, joy riding in stolen cars, and many other forms of
crime and delinquency are traceable to oscillation needs. Like
adults, kids need thrills, excitement, and arousal. They also need to
balance the thrills—to chill out, to relax, to vegetate.

Parents meet important arousal needs by teaching their children (or giving them the opportunity to learn for themselves) how
to turn on to the thrill of competitive sport, to get a rush from
climbing mountains, excelling in school, jamming on a piano, or
pushing their computer skills to new heights. Teaching their children how to shut down, how to relax, and how to get genuine relief
completes the cycle—and sometimes this is the hardest part.

10. TEACH YOUR CHILDREN HOW TO THINK AND ACT DURING TOUGH
    TIMES.

A little preparation goes a long way. One or two simple rehearsals of what to do when your son's or daughter's car breaks down on the highway can substantially reduce the risk of a nontough panic response. Because so much of life is unpredictable and unknown, learning how to think and act in ways that enhance problem-solving is a critical life skill. Tough kids go into tough situations with the feeling "I can handle whatever comes my way."

Teaching children how to solve problems, how not to panic, and how to think things through clearly before acting can make a substantial difference in their ability to control negative arousal. Kids need to know how thinking and acting impacts feelings and emotions. Being prepared for tough times simply means a code of acting and behaving that reinforces personal control.

Obviously, parents who model tough thinking and acting during tough times become the most powerful teachers.

11. IMPART A CORE OF BELIEFS AND VALUES THAT EMPOWER YOUR
    CHILDREN TO TAKE MORE RESPONSIBILITY FOR THEIR OWN TOUGHNESS
    AND HAPPINESS.

Parents who impart a love of life, a passion for living, send a powerful message to their children. No matter how tough life is, there is joy and happiness to be found.

- You can learn to be as tough as you need or want to be. Life is a gift and a privilege and is to be lived to the fullest. Go after it with courage and gusto. Absorb life's hits with poise and resiliency, and move on. Each new day is a new beginning, an unchartered adventure.
- Be kind to yourself and to others, and savor every moment. Life is what you make it and you can make it *big*! Your future is clearly in your own hands. Go for it with toughness and balance and belief in yourself. It's one helluva ride!

12. DON'T ALLOW SIBLING ABUSE.

Low-level conflicts between siblings are a normal part of growing up. However, if serious violence or threats involving weapons occur, or if one child becomes the constant victim of older, stronger, or more aggressive siblings, parents must take firm action to put an end to it.

Don't wait for your children to "grow out of" sibling abuse; the most serious damage is usually done before the age of 12. Without parental intervention, the victimized child is likely to sustain psychological damage of a far more serious and permanent nature than the physical injuries suffered.

Serious conflicts occur more often between the ages of 6 and 12 than in the teens. Stuttering, dangerously low self-esteem, and severe depression are some of the problems traced to excessive sibling abuse in a 1992 study by the University of Michigan's Sandra Graham-Berman. Her study group consisted of white, upper-middle-class college students, indicating that the problem is widespread in our society.

13. TEACH YOUR CHILDREN HOW TO TOUGHEN AND FIND BALANCE IN THEIR LIVES.

Explore ways to get the message across that to get tougher, your children must go beyond their comfort zones. They have to push; they have to stretch themselves beyond their normal limits.

One of the most effective ways is to push yourself, not them. Set the right example—lead from in front, rather than trying to push from behind.

And, once stretched to new limits, you and your children must seek balance by creating powerful waves of recovery and rest. In the symmetry of stress and recovery is found the balance that is vital to all of life.

Work hard—rest equally hard. Make waves, powerful, symmetrical waves. Maximum health, happiness, and productivity are the payoffs.

MEETING NEEDS IS WHERE IT'S AT

All behavior starts making sense when needs are understood. Parents who are successful in teaching their children how to recognize, understand, and fulfill their needs in constructive, healthy ways have taken one of the most important steps they can in producing well-adjusted, tough adults.

Once kids learn to listen and accurately interpret the language of recovery, the more self-understanding they will develop and the better chance they will have of getting their needs met. Connecting feelings and emotions, particularly negative feelings, to unmet needs is a crucial step in effective self-management.

Seems simple enough. Kids eat when they're hungry, sleep when they're tired, and hang out with their friends when they need to belong. Unfortunately, however, when needs are not getting met regularly, messages get distorted, confused, and garbled. That's when deciphering becomes very difficult.

When signals get crossed, kids can start eating to relieve loneliness or boredom, sleeping to relieve depression or guilt, having sex to meet the need to belong, getting into trouble at school to get parents to pay more attention and show more love—the list goes on and on.

Simply put, kids do things they think will meet their needs and tend not to do things that don't. Kids are always looking for ways to find relief—relief from boredom, stress, fear, insecurity, loneliness—all the emotional needs that really scorch keen young appetites and white-hot young emotions. They're also always looking for ways to get a buzz, to get the adrenaline flowing, to spike up, to get high—to beat back boredom and make life sing. If parents don't provide ways to meet those needs, kids will find their own ways. Count on it!

THE JOIN-A-GANG PHENOMENON

As many as 70,000 kids joined gangs to meet their needs in Los Angeles alone. Parents are dumbfounded.

"Why would kids be so stupid? Why would my son ever want to do such a thing? He's a good boy. He's not into violence, hurting people, or crime. It makes no sense!"

Clearly it doesn't make sense from the parents' perspective. But joining a gang becomes completely understandable within the context of unmet needs.

As we learned in Chapter 4 from Maslow's Hierarchy of Needs, safety and security needs are extremely powerful. The fear of being hurt produces massive stress. On the priority list, safety and security needs are near the top.

Kids will do almost anything to get relief. If joining a gang is the only answer, so be it! "I want to get to school alive and make it home in one piece!" Can you blame them? Given the circumstances they are obliged to live in, do they have any intelligent alternative?

During adolescence, the need for belonging and acceptance is also very powerful. Feeling rejection and alienation from one's peers during the fragile adolescent years is deeply painful. "If the only way I can get relief is by joining a gang and taking a few drugs, so be it!"

Next, let's throw in the need to buy food and clothes. Most gang members come from poverty-stricken homes and can't find legitimate employment. The gang promises a job with flexible hours and high wages. "If joining a gang and selling a few drugs is what I have to do to eat and buy clothes, so be it!"

Lastly, let's include the need for relief from boredom. Kids need excitement, challenges, and stimulation. The gang certainly gets the adrenaline flowing. Gangs are anything but boring. "If the only way I can get high is to join a gang and take a few drugs, so be it!"

That's four for four. Kids join gangs because the payoff is big in terms of need fulfillment. The challenge to parents is to find better ways to meet those needs.

26 MORE TIPS ON RAISING TOUGHER KIDS

1. Work on your own toughness every day. Learn the process from the inside. If you're a wimp, you won't be a very believable toughness teacher for your children.

2. Train your children to eat often and light. Get them into the habit of eating something healthy every two or three hours. Teach them to graze, not gorge.

3. Educate your children about nutrition. Get them to read and understand labels on food. Get them into eating and liking healthy foods.

4. Train your children to go to bed early and get up early. Early

to bed and early to rise is the optimal sleep schedule for toughening purposes.

5.   Ensure that your children get eight to nine hours of sleep a night and encourage them to take and enjoy afternoon naps. This will take leadership.

6.   Provide lots of hugs and kisses and affection throughout childhood. Remember, love and affection in the early years are far more important than strictness and discipline.

7.   Start your children exercising as early as possible. Use games, sports, anything to get them moving physically. Your goal is to get them to associate physical activity with fun and excitement. Being more physically fit automatically means tougher.

8.   Expose your children to a wide variety of sports between the ages of 6 and 12. From basketball to soccer and from gymnastics to tennis, let them play. Emphasis should be on fun, not on winning; on developing, not on performing. Team play is preferred over individual competition in the early years, but here again, minimize pressure and maximize fun.

9.   Toughen your children with unconditional, ever-present love, particularly in the early years. It's impossible to overlove children in their first two or three years. Love is the principal mechanism for balancing emotional stress during childhood. Lots of love in the early years builds the foundation for flexibility, responsiveness, strength, and resiliency as adults.

10.   Be responsive to the physical and emotional needs of your children. Meeting needs of children at the right times and in the right ways is what tough parenting is all about.

11.   Learn to properly interpret the language of recovery when the bodies of your children are talking. When your baby cries, is he or she expressing anger, hunger, tiredness, or loneliness? When your sixth-grader starts withdrawing emotionally, is he or she angry, hurt, or afraid? When your 3-year-old throws a temper tantrum, is it out of jealousy, is it to get attention, or is it low blood sugar?

12.   Listen to the needs of your children and learn to separate what's really important from what's not. A child who is angry and negative because his mother wouldn't buy him a toy is one thing. A child who is angry and negative because he feels no one likes him is quite another.

13.   Say no and make it stick when you genuinely feel it's the right

thing, but give your reasons, even if you're saying no to meet your own needs or out of your own anger. If you're angry, give yourself some time to think clearly before you make your decision. "I've thought about it and I've decided you cannot go to the movies tonight because of the way you've been treating me and your sister. Maybe you'll get the message!"

14. Use positive incentives and encouragement to stimulate and motivate. Use fear as a strategy of last resort to keep your children on track and under control.

15. Establish a clear code of ethics, values, and guidelines that become the foundation for everything. The anchors are integrity, honesty, sincerity, cooperation, loyalty, character, faith, and friendship.

16. You get back what you give. Make the four elements of toughness come alive on a daily basis with your children and that's precisely what you'll get back. If toughness is what you want from your children, that's what you've got to model yourself.

17. Be very careful when you start pressuring your children to achieve. For many kids, just a little parental pushing becomes excessive and results in overtraining. Remember, only stress that challenges leads to toughening. If pushing means challenging, you're okay.

18. Teach your children how to make powerful, healthy waves. Learning how to get a healthy high and how to shut down naturally makes unnatural and potentially harmful strategies less attractive or appealing. From sports to mountain climbing and from laughter to yoga, the tools are there to get the chemistry moving.

19. As a parent, you'll naturally try to interest your children in the things that work for you and avoid the things that don't. Remember that your children won't necessarily share your enthusiasms and distastes—what works for you may be poison for them, and vice versa. The important thing is to get your children to find out what works for them. When you identify the right things, use them.

20. Prepare your children for tough times. Use every opportunity you can to train your kids how to think and act when adversity strikes. When the storms of life descend, positive arousal, tough thinking, tough acting, clear thinking, and trained recovery should automatically kick in. When your children are prepared, the storms will leave them tougher and stronger.

21. Constantly encourage your children to express how they feel

and remain open, nondefensive, and accepting whatever they tell you. Teaching your children how to achieve emotional relief through talking means giving them lots of practice. This is particularly true for boys. To get them and keep them talking, you've got to be a great *nonjudgmental* listener. In the context of recovery, feelings are neither right or wrong—they simply are.

22.   Constantly foster independence and self-reliance in your children. Overprotection breeds dependency. Many parents have great difficulty letting go, expanding limits, and increasing freedom as the child grows. The result is always diminished personal growth and toughness. Diminished toughness means your children will have a rougher time when they finally obtain full freedom—or have it thrust upon them by unexpected events.

23.   Teach your children to value their feelings, both positive and negative, and teach them to search for the hidden meanings. Understanding feelings is the first step in getting one's needs met. Feelings are windows to unmet needs, and parents need to help their children make the connection in conscious, thoughtful ways.

24.   Encourage your children to recognize and express feelings of discomfort associated with needs for love, self-esteem, belonging, or intimacy. Only when feelings of insecurity or inadequacy can be identified and understood can relief and new answers be found. So much of adult life is spent trying to protect and cover up perceived weaknesses and fears. Learning in childhood how to access painful feelings and trace them to their source means healthier, less defensive, more balanced adults.

25.   Make toughness in your children a high priority. Talk about it. Read about it. Connect it to their happiness, productivity, and health. Discuss how you get it and how you lose it, the meaning of pain, how to push yourself, and the consequences of pushing too hard. Help your children to relate active and passive toughening, trained recovery, negative and positive arousal, need fulfillment, and wave-making to their own lives.

26.   And, most important, always strive to be as flexible, responsive, strong, and resilient as possible with your children. In other words, be a tough parent—tough in what you expect of yourself and tough in what you expect of them. Do that and you'll raise tough kids who can flourish in tomorrow's tougher world.

13

EDUCATING

TOUGH KIDS:

WHY SCHOOLS FAIL

Go into most classrooms in America and start asking the students, "What do you think about school?" In reply you're likely to hear such words as:

> Dull
> Boring
> Stupid
> Wasted
> Irrelevant
> Unenjoyable
> Nonstimulating

Ask students, "What are your most common feelings during school?" Their answers will probably list some of the following emotions:

Bored	Moody
Tired	Negative
Afraid	Nervous
Annoyed	Unfocused
Stupid	Angry

Tell teachers and administrators about the negative feelings their students have regarding school and it's not likely to come as any great shock or revelation. The students know it. Teachers and administrators know it. Everybody knows it. It seems that it's no surprise to anyone. The impression one gets is that it's normal for kids to dislike school. Hating school is simply a fact of life. School was never meant to be fun. It's a workplace. Students are there to learn, not to have fun.

Tell a coach, however, that his players feel bored, angry, negative, and unmotivated and see what kind of response you'll get, particularly if he is a winning coach or, even better, a professional coach whose job is on the line if the team doesn't perform well. You'd better believe you'll get a vastly different response from what you got when you told teachers and administrators. You'll instantly get his undivided attention.

To coaches who know anything about performance, that's disastrous feedback. Whether teamwide or individual, the news would prompt an immediate investigation into causes and solutions. You'd get action, and lots of questions, like Why? How did it happen? What can be done to change it? Good coaches fully understand how learning and performance are powerfully linked to motivation and attitude. Coaches can cite case after case of how even a single player with a negative attitude has eroded a team's performance potential.

See the reaction you'd get if you told a division head or a production manager that his or her employees are feeling increasingly negative, unmotivated, and angry. Ask an experienced troop commander about the effect of poor morale on the ability of a battalion to carry out its mission. What you'll hear is what you heard from coaches: "This is a serious matter that demands—and will get—immediate attention." You'd get the same response in any arena where learning, training, and performance are important issues.

So why is it different when it comes to school? Why is it that when a child feels negative, bored, unmotivated, or angry about school, no one stirs? Why is it that feeling negative almost seems to be expected in school? It's as if that's the way it's supposed to be. *Negative is normal in school* appears to be the message. Reports of negative attitudes receive little or no attention unless students start causing trouble or failing.

THE SIGNS ARE EVERYWHERE

Chapter 3 of this book explored the concepts of overtraining and undertraining in both life and sport. Do the negative feelings students have during school sound a familiar chord from that chapter? It should. As you recall, feelings of boredom, fatigue, low motivation, low enjoyment, moodiness, negative thinking, and the like are classic signs of *overtraining* and *undertraining*.

And, as we'll come to see and understand, that is precisely the problem with our schools today. Issues of excessive stress, insufficient stress, excessive recovery, and insufficient recovery are at the very core of the problems faced by students today. And the costs for not responding to the messages of overtraining and undertraining are tragically high.

By nearly every measure, our schools are failing. National average scores on standardized exams such as the SAT and ACT continue to decline every year. Our children rank at the bottom of over 15 industrial nations in math, writing, and reading. Our teenage suicide rates are among the highest in the world. Illiteracy rates continue to be high. Crime, violence, delinquency, and drugs have become everyday realities in public schools across America. The signs of failure are everywhere.

TEN WAYS SCHOOLS FAIL

Within the context of the Toughness Training model, schools fail for the following reasons:

1. SCHOOLS FAIL BY NOT IMPROVING THE LEARNING CLIMATE IN THEIR CLASSROOMS.

The ideal climate for performing (IPS) is remarkably similar to the ideal climate for *learning*. For maximum productivity and learning, children should feel excited, eager, happy, and positive about school. They should feel involved, stimulated, and challenged with the learning. Children should feel good about themselves because of school. Like the ideal performing climate, the ideal learning climate means having positively energized, relaxed, calm, happy, and challenged students.

A major part of teacher evaluation should be whether they can consistently sustain this ideal learning climate in their classrooms.

2. SCHOOLS FAIL BY BEING IRRELEVANT AND UNRESPONSIVE TO THE PERCEIVED NEEDS OF STUDENTS.

Bored, angry, negative, tired, and fearful feelings signal unmet needs. All too often, teachers and administrators fail to interpret and respond to expressions of such feelings. Chronically unmet needs—be they mental, emotional, or physical—form the basis of overtraining. Unmet needs mean inadequate recovery. Without adequate recovery, all stress eventually becomes excessive. Irrelevant subject matter and unresponsive teachers inevitably lead to classic overtraining.

3. SCHOOLS FAIL BY NOT USING EXERCISE TO ACTIVELY TOUGHEN STUDENTS.

Most American children today are seriously undertrained physically. Seven hours of inactivity at school followed by five to six hours of motionless TV-watching provide the basis. Only the fortunate few who become involved in interschool competitive sports are spared.

Physical education classes typically lack the frequency, intensity, and focus that leads to toughening. Only through daily rigorous exercise programs for all students, structured for fun and

games, will students learn to use exercise to toughen themselves
and break cycles of linearity and high stress.

Children are desperate for relief from the countless emotional
stressors associated with growing up in today's world. Physical exercise can help bring the needed relief. We must never forget that
if children don't find relief in healthy, constructive ways, they'll get
relief somehow, whether we approve of their method or not.

4. SCHOOLS FAIL BY OVERTRAINING WITH TOO MUCH PRESSURE, TOO
   MUCH HOMEWORK, TOO MANY THREATS, AND TOO MUCH LINEARITY,
   AND NOT ENOUGH FUN, LAUGHTER, AND RECOVERY.

One of the biggest mistakes teachers make is to assume that the
route to accelerated learning is more pushing, more pressure,
more homework, more tests, more discipline, more control. Remember, simply cranking up the volume of stress without balancing
it with recovery leads straight to overtraining. Making first-graders
struggle with homework and pressuring them to perform well on
regular tests do not necessarily accelerate toughness. In fact, without equal attention to fun and recovery, what you'll get is exactly
the opposite—increased alienation, increased anger, boredom, dependency, and fear, all of which are symptoms of overtraining.

5. SCHOOLS FAIL BY MAKING CLASSROOMS OVERLY RIGID, INFLEXIBLE,
   AND CONTROLLING.

Children are separated by age, not according to maturity or readiness to learn a skill. Classrooms are configured in long, straight
rows with communications going one way—forward toward the
teacher. Children are confined to their desks for hours on end, pas-
sively listening to what teachers want them to learn. Although our
knowledge base about child development and learning is greater
than ever before, only rarely do public schools reflect the new understandings.

In the 1960s and 1970s, schools experimented with open education in which students were given maximum freedom and little
structure. Open education was misinterpreted to mean that students could do anything they wanted. Not surprisingly, the movement failed. The reaction we've seen in the 1980s and 1990s is
essentially a "back to basics" return to the failed methods that pre-
ceded open education. Translated, this old-new approach simply

means more homework, more tests, more pressure, more discipline. Neither extreme has produced the desired results. Clearly, the answer must be found elsewhere.

6. SCHOOLS FAIL BY NOT MEETING RECOVERY NEEDS ASSOCIATED WITH FOOD AND NUTRITION.

Most children skip breakfast and by midmorning find themselves energy-deficient and hungry in school because of declining blood sugar levels. When that happens, even the most exciting teacher presentations fail to keep children tuned in. They are increasingly irritable and edgy, and their thoughts turn away from learning toward food and rest.

When lunchtime finally does arrive, they are likely to be served nutritionally deficient foods that are high in fat and simple sugars. School lunches typically consist of easy-to-prepare fried foods such as burgers, fries, hot dogs, tacos, and pepperoni pizza. Seriously lacking are complex carbohydrates in the form of fresh fruits and vegetables, salads, rice, pasta, and whole-grain breads. Most school nutritionists are capable and dedicated professionals, but without the proper financial commitment on the part of the school board, good nutrition can't be provided.

Instead of using lunch to teach students about nutrition, health, and how to achieve maximum recovery benefits from food, schools perpetuate poor eating habits and foster nutritional ignorance. Between discouraging movement and encouraging the consumption of high-fat foods, schools are a major part of the problem. Instead of developing the tougher, leaner, healthier, smarter children America must have to compete in tomorrow's tougher global economy, today's schools are turning out millions of overweight, undereducated softies.

Remember, when recovery needs associated with food and water are not adequately met, nothing else has much meaning. Unstable blood sugar levels mean unstable, weakened learners.

7. SCHOOLS FAIL BY NOT MEETING RECOVERY NEEDS ASSOCIATED WITH OSCILLATION AND MOVEMENT.

Remaining inactive for long periods of time takes tremendous effort and energy for children. A significant number of children simply cannot do it. For many, sitting still is far more tiring and stressful than moving around the classroom. The frontal lobe area of the brain is often immature and slow to develop in children. The frontal lobe plays a major role in curbing arousal and activation.

Oscillation in the classroom for young children means *movement* followed by *brief stillness* followed by *movement* followed by *brief stillness*. As children mature and deepen their capacity for managing stress, periods of stillness can be lengthened. Prolonged stillness is agonizingly boring for most children. Research continues to show that children learn better—they acquire a firmer grasp on more knowledge in less time—when they become active participants in the learning process. Learning by doing is still best. Hands-on is more relevant and far superior to listening for children.

8. SCHOOLS FAIL BY NOT MEETING RECOVERY NEEDS ASSOCIATED WITH SAFETY AND SECURITY.

One of the most disruptive forces attacking classroom learning is crime and violence in the schools. Fear and violence rooted in racial tension, poverty, and drug abuse have become everyday realities for hundreds of thousands of American schoolchildren. Guns, knives, metal detectors, gang warfare, and armed security guards are part of their world, and this is perhaps the greatest single threat to American education.

This is not simply a deplorable problem. Until needs for safety and security are fully met, until schoolchildren can leave home, remain in school, and return home without fear of bodily harm, there can be no realistic hope for significant personal learning, and no substantial improvement in our nation's overall educational effort.

9. SCHOOLS FAIL BY DEMANDING TOO MUCH TOO SOON.

Research in education repeatedly shows that the best way to teach young children is through their natural inclination to play. What may appear like unimportant wasted *play* to an adult is in reality the important *work* of childhood. One of the biggest mistakes schools make is forcing children to work as adults work, too hard and too soon. Demanding more work and less play for younger and younger students does not accelerate meaningful learning. Quite the contrary—this practice seriously erodes the child's natural inclination to learn.

Children's natural drive to learn is amazingly strong and powerful. Schools must nourish this drive, as it is the most precious ingredient in the formula for learning. Children are eager to learn *until we overtrain them* by demanding—earlier and earlier—more work, which automatically means less play.

Pressure to meet performance expectations in the formative years can seriously undermine self-esteem. The effect of early school failure can have serious long-term consequences. When a child's sense of worth and competence is seriously threatened in the early developmental years, the result often is rigidity, defensiveness, unresponsiveness, anger, and negativism in later life.

10. SCHOOLS FAIL BY NOT DIRECTLY TEACHING STUDENTS HOW TO TOUGHEN THEMSELVES FOR THE CHALLENGES OF SCHOOL AND LIFE.

Schools teach reading, writing, and math because—as it's argued—those skills are important in adult life. The same rationale is used for hundreds of other course offerings, from American history to home economics. But how important is it for children to learn how to toughen themselves to meet the myriad challenges they'll certainly encounter in their lifetimes?

How important is it that they learn about recovery, wavemaking, and the consequences of overtraining and undertraining? Expecting children to acquire this critical information on their own or from their parents reveals a lamentable lack of vision. Far too many children find unhealthy answers—not a surprising development when so many come from homes ravaged by poverty, divorce, immaturity, and addiction. In hundreds of thousands of cases, unless the schools take decisive action to break the pattern, it will repeat in generation after generation.

Exposure to toughening concepts should begin as soon as children start school and continue in various forms through high school. Few areas of learning are more central to sustained happiness, productivity, and health than learning how to balance stress and recovery in one's life. Schools must take the lead.

TEN WAYS SCHOOLS CAN TOUGHEN STUDENTS

1. PLACE THE HIGHEST PRIORITY ON THE LEARNING CLIMATE CREATED BY TEACHERS, PARTICULARLY IN THE EARLY GRADES.

Make classrooms more stimulating and more fun. Send a powerful message to teachers that boring classrooms and classrooms dominated by fear will not be tolerated.

Both boredom and fearfulness undermine children's natural love for learning and set the stage for early emotional overtraining. Boredom and fear do not toughen children. Toughening, and the swifter and deeper learning that toughness fosters, takes place when warm and affectionate teachers who sincerely care establish the foundation for flexibility, responsiveness, strength, and resiliency. Once established, in most cases that foundation will last throughout the child's schooling and carry over into later life as well.

2. PLACE THE HIGHEST PRIORITY ON MAKING SCHOOL MORE RELEVANT TO THE PERCEIVED NEEDS OF STUDENTS.

The irrelevancy of school is a major roadblock to toughening. When the expressed needs of students go unmet week after week, year after year, the cycle of stress is chronically perpetuated and the accompanying linearity persistently erodes the toughening process.

3. USE DAILY PHYSICAL EXERCISE TO ACTIVELY TOUGHEN STUDENTS.

A high level of physical fitness should be required of all students throughout the school years. A wide variety of games and physical training exercises should be used to achieve targeted cardiovascular and muscular fitness levels. A major objective of the program should be to teach students to associate physical training with fun and enjoyment. Important also is teaching children how to use exercise to seek constructive relief from stress. Teachers should be strongly encouraged to exercise with the students whenever possible.

4. SERVE ONLY BALANCED, NUTRITIOUS FOODS FOR LUNCH, AND
   CONSTANTLY TEACH STUDENTS ABOUT THE ROLE OF NUTRITION IN
   RECOVERY.

School lunches should conform to the 65 percent carbohydrates, 20 percent fat, and 15 percent protein formula as much as possible. Food should not be fried. Ample quantities of fresh fruit and vegetables should be available daily. Foods high in simple sugars should not be provided. Just as in professional sport, lunch should be thought of as a training table for high-level performance.

Lunchtime must be considered a valuable opportunity to teach students how to assemble nutritious, tasty meals that will maximize energy recovery.

5. SERVE A COMPLEX-CARBOHYDRATE SNACK EVERY 2 TO 2½ HOURS TO
   STABILIZE BLOOD SUGAR.

Students who begin school around 8:00 A.M. should receive a light snack around 10:00, and those remaining past 3:00 P.M. should also be given a light carbo snack. The carbohydrate can be taken either in liquid or solid form. The Tough™ carbohydrate wafer was created specifically for this purpose. The wafer contains 3.3 grams of complex carbohydrate, costs only about ten cents, and tastes like candy to most children. Other options include fruits of all kinds and whole breads, as well as some sport drinks.

6. DO WHATEVER IS NECESSARY TO MAKE SCHOOLS SAFE.

Students should have no fear of being hurt during school, or while going to or from school. Few things can block learning and development more powerfully than this fear. If schools cannot be made safe, then parents must explore other options, including private schools, relocation, or even home learning. This is clearly one of the greatest threats to American education.

7. STIMULATE RATHER THAN PUSH, CHALLENGE RATHER THAN THREATEN,
   PARTICULARLY IN THE EARLY GRADES.

Capitalize on children's natural drive to learn. Be careful not to overtrain young children with too much pressure, too much homework, too much pushing. Exposure to persistent learning stress during the formative years clearly does not toughen children, nor does it accelerate learning. Creating powerful cycles of positive arousal through goal-directed games and play followed by recovery and rest works best.

8. TEACH STUDENTS HOW TO BALANCE THE STRESS OF SCHOOL WITH INTERMITTENT EPISODES OF TRAINED RECOVERY.

Offer toughening classes throughout the school-age years as part of the normal curriculum. Students should be taught how to balance the stress of exams, homework, family, growing up, and socializing with laughter, naps, rest, exercise, and proper eating. The latest research on such things as overtraining and undertraining, sleep, diet, exercise, health, and immune function should be disseminated in creative and dynamic ways. Schools should directly teach children how to think and act under stress to maximize performance output and how to toughen themselves on a daily basis, for these are fundamental life skills.

9. MAKE CLASSROOMS MORE OPEN, FLEXIBLE, AND CHALLENGING, AND LESS CONTROLLING AND CONFORMING, PARTICULARLY IN THE EARLY YEARS.

Rigid, inflexible classrooms produce rigid, inflexible, dependent students. Open classrooms do not mean children get to do whatever they want. Open means flexible, responsive, child-centered—and teaching that's active rather than passive.

10. GET STUDENTS TO MAKE WAVES CONSTANTLY.

Get children moving, get them to be still; get them serious, get them laughing; push them, let them rest; challenge them, let them play; exercise their bodies and let their minds rest; exercise their minds and let their bodies rest; constantly challenge and then recover, challenge and then recover. Keep the juices flowing in both directions in every healthy way possible.

SUMMARY

School leaves many children more passive, dependent, confused, distant, angry, and indifferent while teaching them very little. After 12 long years of daily influence, children leave school unprepared to meet the challenges of adult life. Not only do schools fail to educate children but, equally tragic, they fail to toughen them for life.

America's failed schools are one of the great problems of our times, a problem that poses enormous risks for every American, regardless of age. The public must demand that educational professionals throw off the failed thinking of the past and begin working effectively to breathe new life and vigor into our schools.

14

TOUGHENING

FOR

WOMEN

Most women don't like to think of themselves as tough. To them, "tough" is a male word, suggesting attitudes and actions that are hard, cold, insensitive, even brutal. Football players are tough, boxers are tough, war is tough. In those contexts most women aren't tough, nor do they need to be.

However, when "tough" is taken to mean emotionally flexible, responsive, strong, and resilient, most women are quick to acknowledge that they both want and need toughness.

Women today face a different spectrum of life challenges than men do, but not an easier spectrum. In many respects the challenges to women are sharper and stronger. Consequently, to achieve a high level of productivity, happiness, and health, women must constantly demonstrate toughness—that is, demonstrate flexibility, responsiveness, strength, and resiliency in the emotional, mental, and physical spheres of life.

Though all of this book is for women as well as men, this chapter addresses some of the distinctive challenges women face. There *are* differences between the sexes. Here are ten of them:

1. IN YOUTH, WOMEN HAVE FEWER OPPORTUNITIES TO TOUGHEN THEMSELVES IN COMPETITIVE SPORTS.

This is changing, but the notion that competitive sports are primarily for boys is deeply rooted in this country's cultural past. Not until recently have serious attempts been made to afford girls the same competitive sport opportunities as boys. Denied the use of sport to toughen themselves physically and emotionally, girls are at a distinct disadvantage when they become women and enter the highly competitive world of business.

2. WOMEN HAVE MUCH MORE POWERFUL HORMONAL RESPONSE SYSTEMS THAN MEN.

How different would the world be if men experienced the same powerful hormonal changes associated with menstruation that women must endure every 28 days? How much more effort is required for women to remain positive and emotionally balanced when the premenstrual hormones start to kick in? Maintaining the Ideal Performance State and controlling mood and energy swings become vastly more challenging during peak hormonal periods.

3. WOMEN ARE EMOTIONALLY MORE SENSITIVE THAN MEN.

Nature has equipped women with powerful maternal instincts that naturally deepen their capacity for caring, feeling, and bonding. The hormonal messengers of emotion are more active and complex for women. And since by nature they are more emotional than men, it is even more important for them to achieve emotional toughness.

4. WOMEN ENCOUNTER VASTLY MORE CAREER ROADBLOCKS THAN MEN.

In a male-dominated work force, a woman typically must be much more competent, balanced, and skillful than a man to get the same job. Her emotional flexibility and resiliency will be constantly challenged both in securing and keeping employment commensurate with her talent and skill. To top it off, ambition in a woman is often viewed as overly aggressive, unattractive, or compulsive. It's unfair, unjust, and unconscionable, but women have to be not only more skillful, more competent, and *tougher* to get ahead in their careers, but more diplomatic too.

5. WOMEN EXPERIENCE MORE EMOTIONAL DEPRESSION THAN MEN.

Although the biochemical mechanism is not fully understood, statistics and studies leave no doubt that the incidence of depression is significantly higher among women than among men. This may simply reflect women's more complex hormonal response systems and the greater frustrations, barriers, and challenges that they face. In any case, actively toughening to control depressive cycles and negative mood swings is of special importance to women.

6. WOMEN HAVE A MUCH HIGHER INCIDENCE OF EATING DISORDERS THAN MEN.

Anorexia and bulimia are almost exclusively female disorders. Part of the reason is probably the media-reinforced idea that the perfect female body is a slender one. For some women, protecting themselves against the powerful temptation to achieve the perfect body by compulsive dieting demands great emotional toughness.

7. SOCIETY IS LESS RESPONSIVE TO WOMEN'S NEEDS THAN TO MEN'S.

Women are expected to be less assertive and more dependent, compliant, and self-sacrificing than men. They are therefore less likely to make their needs known and get them met in direct and healthy ways. The persistent nonfulfillment of personal needs perpetuates cycles of unrelieved stress and substantially increases the risk of overtraining.

8. THE BOUNDARIES OF WORK AND NONWORK ARE NOT AS WELL DEFINED FOR WOMEN AS THEY ARE FOR MEN.

For most men the distinction between work and nonwork is easy. Work is simply their job and everything else is nonwork. Women work at their jobs; at home they work at preparing meals, work at raising kids, work on the house, and on and on. Opportunities for recovery breaks, based on work/rest cycles, are less distinct and clear-cut for women, making overtraining more likely.

9. SOCIETY EXPECTS EVERY MOTHER TO BE SUPERMOM, AND PRESSURES MOTHERS TO DO ALL AND BE ALL FOR THEIR CHILDREN.

Personal needs get lost in the guilt-driven urgency to do everything for everyone. Women are more vulnerable than men in this regard because of their powerful maternal instincts. Being a Supermom usually means just being an overtrained regular mom.

10. WOMEN SUFFER FAR MORE SEXUAL HARASSMENT THAN MEN.

Sexual harassment can cause tremendous emotional pain for women. Learning how to prevent it and how to respond to it if it does occur is an important life skill and requires great toughness. The tougher a woman is—emotionally, mentally, and physically— the more in control she will be in the face of sexual harassment.

--- TRACKING THE TOUGH ISSUES ---

The many distinctive challenges women face as they move from childhood through adulthood require great emotional flexibility and strength. Only a few can be addressed in the confines of this chapter. The following five have been selected for consideration here:

- Getting competitive
- Controlling depression
- Controlling PMS
- Losing weight and dieting
- Combating eating disorders

GETTING COMPETITIVE

Deprived of early competitive sport experiences, women often believe that by nature they simply cannot become competitive. Like the usual concept of toughness, the thought of being competitive seems uncomfortable, foreign, and unfeminine. Men are competitive; women are too sensitive and nurturing to be competitive. Many women feel that men don't like tough, competitive women.

In the minds of many women, to be competitive means to be rough, hard, and cold emotionally, and because that's not the way they are or want to be, they deliberately avoid competitive situations altogether. Unfortunately, this avoidance strategy gives their male counterparts in nearly every phase of life a distinct advantage. Males who are less competent, skillful, or experienced will get the break because they have learned how to compete effectively to get what they want.

The first step in getting more competitive is to understand what competition really is. Most women are surprised to learn that competitiveness need have nothing to do with hardness or coldness and everything to do with fun and joy. Being competitive simply means having Ideal Performance State control. It means you can go into competitive situations and experience fun, enjoyment, high positive energy, and confidence.

Good competitors have learned to get the positive juices flowing when they pit themselves against others in pursuit of a goal. Being mean, ruthless, or cold has no relevance whatsoever. Research into competitive skill bears this out.

The notion of "killer instinct" is most unfortunate in sport because it connotes the exact opposite of what we know to be true. "Killer" suggests coldness and ruthlessness, and "instinct" suggests something genetic. Both associations are completely unfounded. Plain and simple, competitiveness is an acquired skill that enables one to enter competitive situations and remain positive, energetic, focused, confident, and optimistic.

Learning to love to compete is learning to get the positive emotions flowing and keep them flowing as you race toward the goal with your fellow competitors. You simply have to develop a sense of fun and get the good juices flowing—and women can learn to do that just as well as men.

HOW TO DEVELOP COMPETITIVE SPIRIT AND POWER

Here are four suggestions to help you strengthen your resolve to compete comfortably and successfully:

1. TAKE THE TIME AND EXPEND THE EFFORT TO BECOME A BETTER COMPETITOR.
Learning how is an important goal; make sure you treat it as such.

2. ATTAIN MASTERY OF YOUR IDEAL PERFORMANCE STATE.
Make gaining that mastery the essential element of your competi-

tive effort. Your most important building blocks for doing that are fun and enjoyment.

3. USE THE TOUGHENING PRINCIPLES YOU'VE LEARNED IN THIS BOOK.
Start by exposing yourself to very mild competitive stress for very short periods of time followed by recovery. This can be done with card playing, bowling, Ping-Pong, and games of all kinds. Your goal is simply to transform feelings of pressure into feelings of fun and enjoyment. As that happens, keep increasing your competitive challenges without getting ahead of your ability to enjoy the pressure.

If feelings of discomfort, insecurity, or low confidence come, employ a recovery strategy, get relief—and then dive right back in. Eventually you'll start loving it!

4. GIVE YOURSELF TIME.
Competitive skills are not learned overnight. IPS control is an important life skill from which you will reap many benefits.

CONTROLLING DEPRESSION

Depression is a pervasive feeling of negative emotion in the form of hopelessness, despair, or sadness. There are two broad categories of depression, situational depression and endogenous depression.

Situational depression occurs in response to a highly traumatic or stressful event such as the death of a loved one, a painful divorce, or the loss of a job. Everyone experiences situational depression from time to time, and it is perfectly normal.

Endogenous depression cannot be linked to any specific event and may, in fact, have a hereditary basis. ("Endogenous" means coming from within rather than from outside.) The rate of endogenous depression in women is almost four times the rate in men. Most authorities today believe that endogenous depression stems from a specific neurochemical imbalance.

Contrary to popular opinion, most endogenous depressions do not result from early parental abusiveness, early deprivation, or early life unhappiness. A characteristic of endogenous depression is its cyclical nature. Accompanied by intense negative feelings, this type of depression affects sleep habits, appetite, and a host of other rhythms associated with stress and recovery.

Two neurotransmitters, norepinephrine and serotonin, are currently thought to be the principal biochemical links in endogenous depression. Of particular interest is the finding that most forms of situational depression remain unaffected by antidepressant medication, but individuals suffering from endogenous depression receive relief as much as 75 percent of the time. Antidepressant medication is targeted specifically to the balance of epinephrine and serotonin. When relief of symptoms occurs in response to such medication, the neurotransmitter imbalance is confirmed.

Control of depression, whether situational or endogenous, is fundamental to happiness, productivity, and health. And since women are much more prone to have problems with depression, they must work especially hard to protect themselves.

TOUGHENING STEPS THAT FIGHT DEPRESSION

1. DETERMINE IF THE DEPRESSION IS SITUATIONAL OR ENDOGENOUS.

Can it be tied to any identifiable stressors? Is it cyclical? As a last resort, can it be controlled with antidepressant medication?

2. KEEP A DEPRESSION LOG.

Monitor the frequency and intensity of the depression on a daily basis. List any factors you suspect contribute to episodes of depression.

3. USE EXERCISE AS YOUR PRINCIPAL STRATEGY FOR BREAKING DEPRESSION.

Both situational and endogenous depression respond positively to exercise. However, some forms of *severe* endogenous depression are not broken by exercise routines and require medication. For most people, however, exercise is the most natural, reliable, convenient, and powerful mood elevator available.

Since exercising may be the last thing you may want to do when you're depressed, talk with friends who will exercise with you or motivate you to get physical.

If possible, take lessons in the sports and exercise activities you get involved in. Lessons help in three important ways:

- You meet people at your same skill level in the sport.
- You gain confidence quicker and enjoy the sport sooner.
- Lessons reduce your chances of accident or injury.

4. REMEMBER THAT DEPRESSION SIGNALS AN UNMET NEED OF SOME KIND.
In the case of endogenous depression, the need is for a better bio-chemical balance; in the case of situational depression, the need is generally for additional emotional recovery. This can be accomplished by talking, exercising, writing, and so on. Remember also that your skills in tough thinking and tough acting can help to move you away from depression toward an empowered state where your needs are more likely to be met.

5. EVALUATE YOUR PROGRESS IN MOOD CONTROL EVERY DAY.
If necessary, seek professional help. Commit yourself to this strug-gle until you have learned to control the depression rather than the opposite. *This is a battle you must win.*

CONTROLLING PMS

Symptoms of PMS (premenstrual syndrome) range from mild irri-tability, moodiness, fatigue, anxiety, and confusion to debilitating depression, disorientation, and withdrawal. PMS can change a woman's total perception of her surroundings and life and can cre-ate difficulties on the job, within the family, and in relationships. Over 90 percent of women worldwide report some kind of emo-tional or physical pain associated with PMS.

Although no definite cause of PMS has yet been confirmed in research, two theories have received considerable attention and some support: the endorphin hypothesis and the serotonin hypoth-esis.

Endorphins produced in the brain, pituitary gland, and other tissues of the body have a morphinelike effect. The release of en-dorphins produces a pleasurable, euphoric mental state. Like mor-phine, endorphins can become highly addictive. Many forms of addictions such as alcoholism and eating disorders are thought to be related to excessive endorphin release.

The endorphin hypothesis is that the symptoms associated

with PMS result from the sudden withdrawal of endorphin that is associated with a woman's menstrual midcycle. Research has confirmed that many women experience a strong endorphin release at ovulation's onset that may be nature's effort to ease ovulation pain. PMS distress is thought to be endorphin withdrawal pain that clears as more endorphins are released with the onset of menstruation.

The serotonin hypothesis is that the primary cause of PMS is a chemical imbalance associated with levels of serotonin. As mentioned earlier, serotonin has been linked to depression and a number of affective disorders. It has been linked to sleep problems, migraine headaches, nausea, and intestinal-tract problems.

As a neurotransmitter, serotonin is a multidimensional chemical messenger that has many links to the symptoms of PMS. The hypothesis essentially holds that low levels of serotonin, both in the brain and circulating, are the culprits. Since serotonin is produced daily from the amino acid L-tryptophan, the theory suggests that diet modification is a major strategy for controlling PMS symptoms.

Researchers at the Massachusetts Institute of Technology found that meals high in carbohydrates facilitate an increase in brain serotonin. The increase in insulin following the ingestion of carbohydrates allows the amino acid L-tryptophan to attach itself to a carrier molecule that can cross to the brain, eventually resulting in increased brain serotonin.

TOUGHENING STRATEGIES FOR PMS

The first step is to decide to be tough enough to beat PMS. Once you've made that decision, the following toughening steps are recommended:

1. ACKNOWLEDGE THAT YOUR PMS SYMPTOMS ARE REAL.
The symptoms are signals your body is sending you; they are not just "in your head."

2. USE DAILY EXERCISE SESSIONS TO REDUCE PMS SYMPTOMS.
If the endorphin hypothesis is correct, the endorphin release occurring during exercise should help to reduce withdrawal symptoms. Many women report exactly that. Two-a-day workouts of 20 to 30

minutes during the most difficult times may be necessary for some women.

3. WATCH YOUR DIET CAREFULLY.

Be sure you're getting most of your calories from carbohydrates (roughly 65 percent). If the serotonin hypothesis is correct, the diet recommended in Chapter 4 to enhance recovery is exactly what is needed to reduce PMS symptoms. Avoid alcohol, caffeine, and chocolate. Instead of overeating, take long tranquil walks.

4. COMMIT ABSOLUTELY TO FINDING THE RIGHT COMBINATION.

Exercise, diet, and tough thinking in combination will lead to PMS control. Convince yourself that you don't have to suffer the agonizing monthly pain associated with PMS. You will not allow this physiological event to in any way compromise your health, productivity, or happiness. You will find the right answers for you! That's a promise!

LOSING WEIGHT AND DIETING

Eating is recovery. Overeating is simply excessive recovery. In terms of calorie intake, stress and recovery in balance means no weight gain or loss. More stress than recovery results in weight loss, and more recovery than stress results in weight gain. The only way to reduce weight is to create an imbalance—expend more calories (stress) than you take in (recovery). Plain and simple, if you want to lose weight, you've got to increase your volume of stress and decrease your volume of recovery.

TOUGHNESS GUIDELINES FOR WEIGHT CONTROL

1. INCREASE YOUR VOLUME OF STRESS THROUGH DAILY EXERCISE.

Interval exercise of low to moderate intensity is the best accelerator of the weight-loss process. High-intensity exercise utilizes energy mostly from blood glucose, while moderate interval exercise converts fat cells into energy.

KEY POINT:

THE ONLY WAY FAT IS LOST IS BY BURNING IT

IN THE MUSCLES. WITHOUT AN APPROPRIATE

EXERCISE COMPONENT, WEIGHT LOSS IS HIGHLY

UNLIKELY, BECAUSE THE VOLUME OF STRESS

CANNOT BE SUFFICIENTLY ELEVATED.

For weight loss, increasing the volume of stress (exercise) is easier and safer for most people than reducing the volume of recovery (the intake of food).

2. MAINTAIN THE TOUGH DIET OUTLINED IN CHAPTER 4.

A diet that is 65 percent carbohydrate, 15 to 20 percent fat, and 10 to 15 percent protein is still your goal. Get the fat out of your diet and you won't end up carrying it around with you. Some fat is necessary and inevitable, but the excessive fat in today's average American diet is the primary culprit.

3. ABSOLUTELY NO FAD DIETS!

Eat the way you are going to eat for the rest of your life or you'll simply gain all the weight back when you go off your diet. Make your diet healthier, not crazier. Fad diets simply undermine recovery and lead to failure and discouragement.

4. NEVER LOSE MORE THAN TWO OR THREE POUNDS A WEEK.

More weight loss than that is *overtraining!* When you overtrain, all the painful symptoms of excessive stress start appearing—fatigue, depression, irritability, moodiness, and so on. These are important warning signals. If you ignore messages of pain, the serious consequences of overtraining can suddenly become a reality. Losing weight too quickly also causes muscle loss. You want to lose fat, not muscle.

5. EAT OFTEN AND EAT LIGHTLY.

This is critical. No fasting, no starvation diets. Dramatically reducing recovery simply causes the body to gear down and function on fewer calories. As soon as you resume normal caloric intake levels, your more efficient body will gain weight more quickly than before. Fasting simply teaches the body how to store fat efficiently.

6. REDUCE CALORIC INTAKE SLIGHTLY, BUT KEEP YOUR BLOOD SUGAR LEVEL STABLE THROUGHOUT THE DAY.

Eat regularly and never go longer than two hours without some form of food intake. The more overweight you are, the more often you should take in calories. This will mean no big meals and lots of low-fat, low-calorie, healthy snacks.

7. CUT BACK—BUT DON'T NECESSARILY ELIMINATE FAVORITE FOODS THAT ARE UNHEALTHY.

Giving up foods you love simply magnifies their importance in your mind. Eat them, enjoy them, but eat less of them. Eating slowly helps prevent overeating.

8. READ, READ, READ.

Get into the habit of reading labels and understanding the language of nutrition. Knowing that one gram of fat has twice as many calories as one gram of carbohydrate is critical information in balancing stress and recovery.

9. USE EXERCISE AS YOUR PRIMARY WEIGHT-LOSS STRATEGY.

The calories you burn during exercise are not the critical factor in weight loss; the changes in body chemistry and metabolism that accompany exercise are more important. Proper exercise also increases muscle mass, which is where calories get burned.

10. DISTINGUISH BETWEEN HUNGER NEEDS AND EMOTIONAL NEEDS.

Eat to satisfy nutrition needs; meet your emotional needs in other ways. Keep in mind that exercise can help you lose weight and give you emotional relief at the same time.

COMBATTING EATING DISORDERS

Two well-publicized eating disorders are anorexia nervosa and bulimia. Some researchers estimate that as many as 4 percent of the general population suffers from bulimic problems and between 1 and 2 percent from anorexia.

Bulimia and anorexia are considered diseases of similar type and origin. Because they afflict mostly women and occur in much greater frequency in specific social contexts, the importance of environmental factors in their development is strongly supported.

Examples are the higher incidence of both anorexia and bulimia among female models, dancers, gymnasts, and tennis players. Extreme social pressure regarding beauty, size, and marketability clearly influences the incidence of both diseases.

The dominant symptom in anorexia is the feeling of being fat even though there is no basis in reality for the feeling. An anorexic can look like a skeleton and still argue that she is too fat. Obsessive fears and thoughts about food are commonplace in anorexic thinking.

The dominant symptom in bulimia is binge eating followed by deliberate vomiting. Bulimics can show fluctuations in weight of more than ten pounds because of the alternating fasts and binges. Both bulimics and anorexics often suffer considerable depression and guilt regarding their behavior and their perceived failure to meet expectations. Both disorders can tragically lead to death from cardiac arrest caused by electrolyte imbalance. As many as 25 percent of all anorexics are involved in bulimia.

The exact causes of both disorders still remain largely speculative, but the most plausible explanation seems to be a combination of social factors and brain chemistry. Here again, we see evidence of an endorphin connection. Anorexics have higher endorphin levels than the general population; this suggests that endorphin release has been conditioned to occur with starvation. What anorexics seem to experience with food denial is not pain but pleasure. Fasting becomes chemically addictive.

A similar rationale can be used for bulimics. Purging becomes addictive because of associated pleasurable endorphin release.

Purging and fasting also create powerful waves of energy expenditure and energy recovery. The alternating rhythms so typical of bulimia clearly force body chemistry to oscillate. Remember, if individuals can't find natural, healthy ways to make waves, they'll meet the need somehow.

──────── **TOUGHENING TACTICS AGAINST ANOREXIA AND BULIMIA** ────────

Here are some suggestions to help prevent and conquer the two most dangerous eating disorders:

1. SEEK PROFESSIONAL HELP IMMEDIATELY.

These are dangerous disorders. If you suspect a problem with yourself or a loved one, particularly if the concern is anorexia, seek professional help. Because anorexics have strong denial and self-deception tendencies, outside progressive intervention is necessary. Bulimics are keenly aware of their problem and often will seek help on their own, or respond positively to suggestions to do so. Anorexics are typically very defensive and resistant to outside intervention.

2. RESIST THE TEMPTATION TO USE FOOD TO MEET EMOTIONAL NEEDS.

Overeating when depressed and fasting to relieve the guilt set the stage for the anorexic/bulimic mechanism to kick in.

3. DON'T ALLOW SOCIETAL PRESSURES TO MAKE YOU OBSESSIONAL ABOUT YOUR LOOKS OR WEIGHT.

Heighten your awareness of the pressures working against you and use tough thinking to be sure you don't become a victim. Never toy with anorexic or bulimic behavior. The stakes are simply too high.

4. RESIST FAD DIETS OF ALL KINDS.

Fad diets change your perception of food and stimulate obsessive behavior. If you need to lose weight, your safest formula for success is simply this:

- Increase your energy expenditure with low to moderate exercise.
- Reduce caloric intake slightly by simply eating smaller portions of your regular, healthy diet and reducing the amount of fat in your diet.

5. LEARN TO MEET YOUR NEEDS FOR OSCILLATION WITH HEALTHY WAVES.

Get the juices flowing and the endorphins moving from exercise so that eating disorders never get a foothold.

KEY POINT:

ANOREXICS AND BULIMICS OFTEN BECOME OBSESSIVE ABOUT

EXERCISE AS WELL AS ABOUT FOOD. SIMPLY RECOMMENDING

THAT INDIVIDUALS SUFFERING FROM THESE DISEASES SHOULD

INCREASE THEIR EXERCISE CLEARLY IS *NOT* APPROPRIATE.

WHEN OBSESSIVE EATING BEHAVIOR TEAMS UP WITH OBSESSIVE

EXERCISE, LITTLE TIME REMAINS. PROMPT INTERVENTION IS REQUIRED

TO SAVE THE PERSON'S LIFE.

6. ANTIDEPRESSANT MEDICATION CAN BE VERY HELPFUL IN BREAKING THE
BULIMIC CYCLE FOR SOME PEOPLE.

Because bulimics often suffer considerable cyclical depression that triggers their binges, reducing the depression can help break the destructive pattern. Unfortunately, no medication has been found to be useful in treating anorexia.

SUMMARY

Women face special challenges that require special toughness. Violence and crime against women such as rape and sexual harassment, eating disorders, career discrimination, depression, and cyclical hormone release are just a few examples. The energy expenditure demands on women today often exceed those on men, yet many more toughening opportunities naturally exist for men than for women.

Today's world is also more responsive to the needs of men than women. For women to achieve maximum levels of productivity, happiness, and health, they have to work harder and smarter; they must be *tougher* than their male counterparts. That simply means that women must seize every opportunity they can to toughen or the reality of overtraining will most certainly strike. Fortunately, the gender inequities are changing, but life goes on and needs must be met now.

Blocked or unfulfilled needs perpetuate cycles of stress and linearity. Women must tune into their bodies, read their needs accurately, and respond. Healthy responses bring harmony and balance. Unhealthy ones bring disorder, unhappiness, and disease. Toughening for women is a must!

15

IT AIN'T

OVER TILL

IT'S OVER!

Toughening for life is forever. Athletes stop training when they retire from *sport*. Training for life toughness must continue until we retire from *life*. Maximum productivity, happiness, and health is the goal in whatever stage of life time's swift passage puts us.

No matter where you are on the scale of toughness, you can and probably need to train to get tougher. Simply agreeing that this is true won't accomplish anything, nor will wishing to get involved in a toughening program. Toughening won't take place unless you do four things:

1. Commit to becoming a healthier, happier, more productive person through Toughness Training;
2. Make the necessary adjustments in your routine that will permit you to devote time and energy to toughening on a daily basis;
3. Monitor your progress in an organized way;
4. Get started right away.

This final chapter details a very simple yet powerful system for monitoring your progress so that you can keep the toughening process moving forward. The only sure way to accelerate our toughness is to directly train for it. To reach our highest potential—our happiest, healthiest, most productive state—we all must go into training and keep training for toughness as long as the wonder of life persists.

It's not a grim prospect. On the contrary, your enthusiastic, joyful, and permanent participation in the Toughness Training for Life program guarantees that your toughened self will enjoy a far richer, more satisfying and exciting life and career than your nontough self could achieve. Moreover, when time begins to afflict your nontough contemporaries with the infirmities of age, your Toughness Training will give you many more years of healthy, happy, productive life. Even if you're at that stage now, the Toughness Training for Life program can help you slow the aging process and even reverse many features of it.

But none of these great things happens by itself. You must start the program and keep it going. It doesn't have to be hard; leaping instantly into the total Toughness Training program isn't essential, particularly if you're a nonexerciser with eating habits that could be improved.

All you really have to do is make a beginning today, and then do a little more on each tomorrow. Change at least one small item of your life-style right now—for example, choose fresh orange juice over a sugary soft drink.

Continue to move into Toughness Training at your own pace—as rapidly as you can but without overwhelming yourself with withdrawal discomfort, stiffness from pushing into exercise too quickly, and heavy stress from revising too much of your life too fast.

Remember, your body likes slow and easy changes, and so do your mind and personality. Your incredibly complex biological systems need time to adapt; make it easy on yourself by giving them that necessary time. You spent your whole life getting into whatever shape you're in now; allow yourself at least a reasonable time to get into the toughened state you want. But don't stall. You can be as tough—that is, as happy, healthy, and productive—as you choose to be. This chapter gives you a system for doing it.

THE TOUGHNESS TRAINING FOR LIFE
CONTROL SYSTEM

The Toughness Training Control System has four components:

1. A daily training log
2. A weekly goal-setting program for toughening
3. A periodic stress/recovery check
4. A 12-week summary page

THE DAILY TRAINING LOG

If you want to get better at something, you've got to track it. Athletes are well aware of the value of training logs. The daily log shown in Figure 15.1 allows you to tune in to the critical variables involved in Toughness Training.

Use the categories listed in the log to get started. Eventually you should create your own training categories that best fit your personal toughness needs. Completing the log takes only about six minutes a day. Each of the training categories is discussed below.

1. *Interval aerobic exercise.* Simply record the approximate time spent today doing intervals within your aerobic zone. A maximum of 80 percent of your cardiorespiratory exercise should be of this kind. The ideal length of exercise for general life toughening is 20 to 30 minutes. Two 30-minute sessions are recommended over a single 60-minute one. If you want or need to work out more than 30 minutes, build in a minimum of two to three hours of recovery between workouts.

2. *Interval nonaerobic exercise.* Simply record the approximate time spent today doing intervals below or above your aerobic zone. Approximately 20 percent of your cardiorespiratory exercise can be above or below your aerobic zone. Only experienced, healthy, well-conditioned exercisers should do waves above their aerobic limits. Check with your physician.

3. *Curl-ups.* Record the number of curl-ups you've done for the day. Your *ultimate* goal is between 150 and 200 a day in sets of 25. Start slowly.

DAILY TRAINING LOG
(Let Me Count the Waves)

	MON	TUE	WED	THU	FRI	SAT	SUN
1. Interval aerobic exercise (time)							
2. Interval nonaerobic exercise (time)							
3. Curl-ups (no.)							
4. Strength training (time)							
5. Stretching (yes/no)							
6. Diet (A–F grade)							
7. Number of meals (often & light)							
8. Quantity of sleep (hours)							
9. Quality of sleep (1–10)							
10. Time to bed/time up							
11. Nap (yes/no)							
12. Lowest & highest pulse for today							
13. Overall volume of stress (1–10)							
14. Quantity of recovery (time)							
15. Quality of recovery (1–10)							
16. Tough thinking (A–F)							
17. Tough acting (A–F)							
18. Negative arousal control (A–F)							
19. Waves of strong positive emotion (no.)							
20. Stress /recovery balance (1–10)							
21. Felt energy, motivation, fun (1–10)							
22. Happy (1–10)							
23. Productive (1–10)							
24. Healthy (1–10)							
25. Got tougher today (yes/no)							

Figure 15.1

4. *Strength training.* Record the amount of time you spent working with machines, free weights, or flexible tubing. Keep a separate log on the number of repetitions, amount of weight, and number of sets. Remember to train a specific muscle group every other day, not daily.
5. *Stretching.* Simply record the number of stretches you completed for the day. If none were completed, write "no."

6. *Diet.* Grade your diet, using the same grading system your teachers did in school—A for excellent, B for good, C for average, D for poor, and F for failure. Judge your diet in terms of the criteria set forth in Chapter 4.

7. *Number of meals.* Record the number of meals you eat during the day. Your goal is four or more light meals. A whole-wheat snack and some fruit would be an example of a meal.

8. *Quantity of sleep.* Record the total number of hours of sleep during the night. Your goal is seven to eight hours daily.

9. *Quality of sleep.* Use the 1–10 scale to evaluate the quality of your sleep. A 1 means the lowest-quality sleep, a 10 the best.

10. *Time to bed/time up.* Record the time you went to bed and the time you got up. Your goal is to be as consistent as possible, particularly during stressful times. For most people, going to bed early and getting up early is the best rhythm.

11. *Nap.* If you took a nap today, record the length of time. If you took no nap, write "no."

12. *Lowest and highest pulse for today.* Take your pulse first thing in the morning to get your lowest pulse; also record your highest pulse achieved during exercise for the day.

13. *Overall volume of stress.* Estimate the total amount of mental, emotional, and physical stress you experienced today using the 1–10 scale. A 1 is the lowest level of stress possible, a 10 the highest.

14. *Quantity of recovery.* Estimate the total amount of time you spent today involved in active or passive rest activities. See Chapter 4 for details.

15. *Quality of recovery.* Estimate the value of the recovery activities in terms of balancing stress. Use the 1–10 scale; a 1 means no recovery value and a 10 means the highest recovery value.

16. *Tough thinking.* Estimate your success at thinking tough today, using the A–F scale. Refer to Chapter 10 for details.

17. *Tough acting.* Estimate your success at acting tough today, and record it using the A–F scale. Refer to Chapter 9 for details.

18. *Negative arousal control.* Estimate your success today in controlling the flow of negative energy—that is, fear and anger. Use the A–F scale.

19. *Waves of strong positive emotion.* Count the number of emo-

tional highs you experienced today—such things as enjoying a sunset, a great run, a laugh with your child. Many things can produce powerful positive waves. Set goals to experience at least two joyful highs each day.

20. *Stress/recovery balance.* Using the 1–10 scale, estimate how much balance you achieved today in terms of stress and recovery. A 1 is no balance and a 10 is perfect balance.

21. *Felt energy, motivation, fun.* Estimate how successful you were today in sustaining feelings of high positive energy, using the 1–10 scale. A 1 means no success and a 10 means total success.

22. *Happy.* Estimate the extent to which you felt happy today using the 1–10 scale. A 1 is no happiness and a 10 is complete happiness.

23. *Productive.* Estimate the extent to which you were productive today, using the 1–10 scale. A 1 is nonproductive and a 10 is peak performance.

24. *Healthy.* Estimate the extent to which you are physically healthy today using the 1–10 scale. A 1 is seriously sick in the hospital, and a 10 is feeling great and completely healthy.

25. *Got tougher today.* Did you push yourself beyond your normal limits today and experience the discomfort of stress that toughens? If you did, give yourself a big yes! If not, give yourself a no.

SETTING WEEKLY GOALS FOR TOUGHENING

At the beginning of each week, select two goals you will work toward during the week. If you wish, you can keep the same goal or goals for several weeks at a time. New goals, however, bring new insights and focus. If you're having trouble with a goal, give yourself a break and come back to it in later weeks. Here are just a few goals you can choose among:

Diet

- Less fat
- More complex carbohydrates
- More frequent meals
- No late meals
- Labels checked before you buy food
- Improved understanding of nutritional science

Recovery

- Increased volume of recovery for the week
- Better sleep consistency
- Afternoon naps
- More active rest
- More passive rest
- More fun times
- Better recovery skills emotionally, such as writing, talking, exercising
- Improved body listening
- Improved understanding of negative emotion
- Improved need recognition and fulfillment

Getting Tougher

- Pushing yourself to become tougher
- Responding better to the ringing phone
- Improved IPS control
- Improved tough-thinking skills
- Improved tough-acting skills
- Increased volume of stress for the week
- Improved body language—look of confidence
- Improved competitiveness
- Learning to respond to adversity with challenge
- Better mistake management
- Improved PMS control
- Improved depression control

Flexibility

- Improved mental flexibility skills
- Improved emotional flexibility skills
- Improved physical flexibility skills

Strength

- Improved mental strength
- Improved emotional strength
- Improved physical strength

Resiliency

- Improved mental resiliency
- Improved emotional resiliency
- Improved physical resiliency
- Improved negative arousal control

WEEKLY REVIEW

At the end of each week, review what you've done to improve in the areas where you set your two weekly goals. By paying special attention to food labels during the week or by reading two articles on nutrition, you moved closer to your goals for that week. In a sense, your weekly goals become special themes in your life for that seven-day period. Simply focusing your attention on these issues leads to new changes.

There are no absolute limits to be met with your weekly goals, only a commitment to focus considerable energy and attention to the issue for seven days. What you want is the personal acknowledgment that this is an important area of learning and growth for you and that for the week it will receive a high priority in your life. The more time you think or write about your goal during the week, the greater the potential for real change.

Display your weekly goals in a prominent place so you will see them many times during the day.

PERIODIC STRESS/RECOVERY CHECKS

In many ways, balancing stress and recovery is like balancing a checkbook. Stress is writing checks and recovery is making deposits. It's much easier to write checks than it is to deposit money. For most, it's much easier to expend energy than it is to recapture it. Chronically spending more money than we deposit eventually means financial ruin. As we learned in Chapter 3, chronically expending more energy than we recapture can be equally disastrous.

The following system for checking the balance of stress and recovery in your life uses numbers just as your checkbook does. Rather than tracking dollars, however, we track units of stress and units of recovery. Ten units of stress must be balanced by ten units of recovery.

Obviously, the numbers are only estimates, but experience has shown that this approach can be extremely helpful in understanding and finding balance. Complete the stress check and the recovery check daily for seven days. This should be done every four to six weeks to sample how you're doing. It is also particularly helpful to complete the stress/recovery check during highly stressful times.

Your goal is to match units of recovery with units of stress on a daily basis. If one day or week your stress scores are quite high compared to recovery scores, your objective is to increase recovery units as soon as possible. A daily stress score of 19 and a recovery score of 18 reflects great balance. Discrepancies of more than 3 units on a daily basis and more than 10 units on a weekly basis deserve your special attention. Obviously, chronic overspending leads to trouble. The summary page (Figure 15.2) enables you to summarize your daily and weekly totals and keep them for quick future reference.

Remember, the higher your stress scores, the more important energy recovery activities become.

STRESS CHECK

1. Quantity of work
    (time working today)   **Hours**

2. Intensity of work
   (how hard you worked)   **3,2,1,0**
   INTENSITY: High 3, Medium 2, Low 1, None 0

3. Intensity of emotional stress associated with work
   (amount of anger, frustration, or nervousness
   during work)   **3,2,1,0**
   STRESS: High 3, Medium 2, Low 1, None 0

4. Travel stress
   (amount of time traveling today)   **Hours**

5. Quantity of physical training
   (no. of hours of running, weight-lifting,
   stretching, etc. today)   **Hours**

6. Intensity of physical training
   (how hard you worked)   **3,2,1,0**
   INTENSITY: High 3, Medium 2, Low 1, None 0

7. Intensity of home-life stress
   STRESS: High 3, Medium 2, Low 1, None 0   **3,2,1,0**

8. Intensity of other stress
   (health, financial, etc.)   **3,2,1,0**
   STRESS: High 3, Medium 2, Low 1, None 0

TOTAL HOURS (PHYSICAL)	**TOTAL INTENSITY (EMOTIONAL)**

- If you smoked 1 to 10 cigarettes, *add 2 points* to your total stress units.
- If you smoked more than 10, *add 3 points* to your total stress units.
- If you drank 3 to 6 oz. of alcohol, *add 2 points* to your total stress units.
- If you drank more than 6 oz., *add 4 points* to your total stress units.

TOTAL HOURS (Physical Stress)	+ **TOTAL INTENSITY (Emotional Stress)**	= **TOTAL DAILY STRESS UNITS**

RECOVERY CHECK

1. Sleep (quantity)   _____
   More than 7 hours = + 4
   5–7 hours = + 2
   Less than 5 hours = +.5

2. Sleep (consistency)   _____
   To bed and up within 30 minutes of normal
   sleep time
   Yes = + 2
   Almost = + 1

3. Nap   _____
   30 minutes to 1 hour = + 2
   Less than 30 minutes = + 1

4. Rest (active—walking, golf, biking, etc.)   _____
   More than 1 hour = + 2
   30 minutes to 1 hour = + 1
   Less than 30 minutes = +.5

5. Rest (passive—reading, movies,
   TV, music, etc.)   _____
   More than 1 hour = + 2
   30 minutes to 1 hour = + 1
   Less than 30 minutes = +.5

6. Relaxation exercise   _____
   (meditation, breath control, yoga, massage)
   More than 1 hour = + 2
   30 minutes to 1 hour = + 1
   Less than 30 minutes = +.5

7. Diet (number of meals)   _____
   4 or more light meals = + 3
   2 to 3 meals = + 1

8. Diet (healthy meals—light, fresh,   _____
   low-fat, complex-carbohydrate-centered)
   Yes = + 3
   Almost = + 1

9. Fun times today   _____
    Feel today was a fun day = + 2

10. Quantity of personal free time·   _____
    1 or more hours = + 2
    30 minutes to 1 hour = + 1

                    TOTAL RECOVERY UNITS _____
                    (Maximum = 24 points)

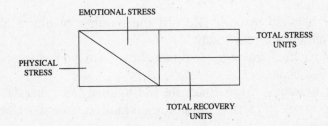

WEEKLY STRESS/RECOVERY SUMMARY
(12 Weeks)

WEEK OF	MON		TUE		WED		THU		FRI		SAT		SUN		TOTAL

Figure 15.2

───────── **CATEGORIES FOR THE STRESS CHECK** ─────────

1. *Quantity of work.* Record the total number of hours you spent working today.
2. *Intensity of work.* Estimate how hard you worked today using a 0–3 scale. A 0 is nothing and a 3 is high intensity.
3. *Intensity of emotional stress associated with work.* Estimate how much emotional stress you experienced today with your work in terms of negative arousal (anger, fear, frustration). Use the 0–3 scale.
4. *Travel stress.* Record the amount of time traveling today. Travel is just as stressful as or even more stressful than regular work for most people.
5. *Quantity of physical training.* Record the number of hours of physical training you did today.
6. *Intensity of physical training.* Estimate how hard you worked, using the 0–3 scale.
7. *Intensity of home-life stress.* Estimate the intensity of home-life *relationship* stress in terms of spouses, children, friends. Use the 0–3 scale.
8. *Intensity of other stress.* Estimate the intensity of other home-related stress such as health, financial, and so on. Use the 0–3 scale.

───────── **CATEGORIES FOR THE RECOVERY CHECK** ─────────

Ten categories are used in estimating the total volume of recovery for a 24-hour period. They are all self-explanatory and therefore will not be listed here. The maximum number of recovery units one can earn in a 24-hour period is 24.

When convenient, simply transfer the totals to the summary page shown as Figure 15.2. It has space for 12 weeks.

MAINTAINING THE SYSTEM

The daily training log takes only a few minutes to complete each day. Your weekly goal-setting program will also require only a few minutes of your time weekly. The stress/recovery check takes 10 to 15 minutes a day and is done only every four to six weeks.

The Toughness Training Control System outlined here provides a powerful way to keep your personal toughening program alive and growing. It isn't time-consuming, and the few minutes you spend each week keeping it up will be amply repaid by your more rapid progress.

Make keeping the Control System fun. Never agonize over the values you assign; make quick decisions without worrying about how consistent you're being. Your evaluations will vary more at first than later. Keep on recording your progress; you'll find that it's a terrific way to motivate yourself to keep on getting tougher.

At a minimum, get into the habit of keeping the daily log. You'll never regret it.

THE TOUGHENING MODEL:
A FINAL QUESTION & ANSWER SUMMARY

Q: What is the meaning of stress and recovery?

Expending energy is stress and recapturing energy is recovery. Everything we do has energy expenditure and energy recovery properties. Once energy is expended it must be eventually recaptured to sustain optimal physiological and psychological health and balance.

Energy expenditure (stress) as well as energy recovery (rest) can occur physically, mentally, and emotionally.

Too much stress or too much recovery creates conditions of imbalance. The greater the imbalance, the greater the potential dysfunction in terms of reduced productivity, happiness, and health.

Q: What is the meaning of toughness?

Toughness is a measure of health and is evidenced specifically in terms of increases in flexibility, responsiveness, strength, and resiliency. Increases in toughness can occur physically, mentally, and emotionally.

Q: Why are emotions so important in the Toughening Model?

Emotions basically run the show in both sport and life. The right emotions free and empower us, and the wrong emotions trap and defeat us. Understanding the meaning of emotion and learning how to control the flow of emotion during special times represent critical life skills.

The reason emotion is so powerfully linked to such things as productivity and health is its connection to physiological arousal. Emotions are biochemical events which can profoundly influence every sphere of physiological and psychological functioning.

Q: *How are emotions connected to stress and recovery?*

Emotions and feelings are body talk reflecting the balance of stress and recovery at any given time. Positive emotional states and particularly empowering states such as enthusiasm, passion, high motivation, challenge, and so on reflect stress/recovery balance.

Negative emotional states and disempowering feelings such as helplessness, depression, fatigue, fearfulness, and so on reflect stress/recovery imbalance.

Q: *How does toughening occur?*

Toughening occurs only in response to progressively increasing levels of stress. To toughen is to expand one's capacity for effectively coping with stress. Toughening physically, mentally, or emotionally can be achieved only by exposure to increasing stress in those areas.

Q: *How does weakening occur?*

Weakening occurs as a response to both too little and too much stress. Protection from stress results in progressive weakening as does exposure to excessive stress. To weaken is to decrease one's capacity for effectively coping with stress. Weakening can occur physically, mentally, and emotionally.

Q: *How important is recovery?*

Without recovery, all stress becomes excessive. Increasing the volume and quality of recovery is essential during periods of high stress. Adequate sleep, proper nutrition, and sufficient rest are fundamental during the toughening cycle to prevent overtraining.

Q: *What are the characteristics of the healthy, toughened person?*

Toughened persons possess the ability to spike great peaks of energy expenditure followed by powerful troughs of energy recovery. They are constantly oscillating and making waves of stress and recovery mentally, physically, and emotionally. Toughened persons remain flexible, responsive, strong, and resilient under stress and operate predominantly from a positive emotional state. They are skillful at getting their needs met in healthy ways and are very proficient at interpreting and responding to the stress/recovery needs of the body. Toughened persons have a great capacity for coping with stress and can readily access empowering emotional states.

Q: *How do we know if the stress we're experiencing is getting us tougher, simply maintaining our current toughness, or weakening us?*

When stress becomes excessive physically, mentally, or emotionally, the body responds by sending messages of pain. Pain is a signal to stop or weakening will occur. Pain in the physical realm is familiar and obvious to most people. Pain in the psychological realm is sent via the negative emotions. Intense anger, fear, frustration, depression, sadness, boredom, etc., are analogous to intense pain in the physical body and serve the same purpose.

To ensure that we are toughening rather than weakening in response to stress we must constantly monitor body talk for messages of discomfort or pain. Discomfort is a signal to pay attention and is the most common message sent while toughening is occurring. To toughen, we must push beyond our normal limits. This is always accompanied by feelings of discomfort. The feelings are clearly not pleasant, but they aren't really painful either. We're simply beyond our normal comfort zone.

No discomfort or no pain in response to stress is a signal we're experiencing normal life stress which will simply maintain our current levels of toughness. Plain and simple, if we want to get tougher, we've got to take on more stress and get uncomfortable for a while.

Q: *How do stress and recovery relate to need fulfillment?*

The urge associated with a need is stress and fulfillment of the urge is recovery. Understanding our needs and fulfilling those needs in healthy, direct ways promotes stress/recovery balance.

Q: *Must we create additional stress in our lives to get tougher?*

We can use normal life stress to toughen ourselves, particularly during periods of crisis and adversity. Tough times actually represent opportunities for getting tougher. Remember, if you don't have any stressful times, you're probably getting weaker. Using normal life stress to toughen is called passive toughening.

Actually seeking greater stress to accelerate the toughening process is an important strategy called active toughening. Deliberately increasing the volume of stress in our lives by exercising, taking on new challenges, adding responsibilities, etc., is an indispensable part of the training process.

Q: *How can we prevent times of high stress from weakening us?*

We can prevent the sudden storms of life from weakening us by doing the following things:

1. Increase the frequency and volume of recovery. Eat, sleep, and rest according to a very precise schedule.
2. Restructure the way we think about the stressful event or period so as to decrease negative arousal. Try to see the crisis as an opportunity to grow, to get tougher, and to learn more about ourselves. Perceiving the situation as a challenge rather than a threat significantly reduces energy expenditure levels.
3. Physically act in ways that suggest we are not under great stress. Show confidence, calmness, courage, and poise on the outside. This reduces negative arousal and overall energy expenditure.

Q: *How much stress must we expose ourselves to in order to maintain our current levels of toughness?*

Great toughness requires that a high level of stress be maintained to prevent weakening. The volume of stress required to maintain our toughness depends completely on our level of toughness. The tougher we are, the more stress we need to experience to maintain current levels.

Q: *If we get tougher physically, will it have an effect mentally or emotionally?*

Increases in toughness in one of the three areas will result in increases in toughness in all areas. The mental, emotional, and physical realms are so intimately connected that when we impact one, we will have some influence on all three.

The reverse is also true. When one of the three starts to weaken, all three are affected.

Q: *How do we know that we have too much recovery? Are there signals of too much rest?*

Absolutely. Too much stress and too much recovery are often signaled by similar feelings of pain. Low motivation, apathy, depression, boredom, fatigue, etc., occur at extremes.

Q: *What does it mean to think tough?*

It simply means thinking and imaging in ways that reduce negative arousal and stimulate effective problem solving and positive action. Tough thinking leads to empowering emotions under pressure.

Q: *What does it mean to act tough?*

It simply means acting on the outside the way we want and need to feel on the inside to perform at our peak. Acting tough stimulates empowering emotions under pressure.

Q: *How can we prepare for the tough times that are certain to come into our lives?*

We must use every day to train to get tougher. Each day of our life is another opportunity to become more flexible, responsive, strong, and resilient.

Q: *How can we gain more control over how we feel during stressful times?*

We must train to become more disciplined in how we think and act as stress increases. Thinking and acting directly connects to our emotional response patterns. Sloppy, negative thinking and acting virtually guarantee loss of control emotionally.

Q: *Should we freely express negative emotions when they occur?*

The suppression of negative emotions during performance is generally performance enhancing. The expression of negative emotions during performance does represent a form of recovery but often stimulates disempowering emotions and strengthens undesirable habits which erode Ideal Performance State control.

The expression of negative emotion outside of the performance context facilitates recovery and is important in establishing stress/recovery balance.

Q: *What is the meaning of negative emotions?*

Negative feelings and emotions signal unmet needs. Intense negative feelings reflect strong unmet needs and vague, nonintense negative feelings reflect weaker ones.

Permanently blocking negative feelings prevents our needs from getting met. Meeting important needs quickly and directly eliminates the need for intense psychological pain in the form of depression, anger, fear, etc., to get our attention.

Learning to understand and properly interpret the way in which negative emotions relate to unmet needs, as well as separating important needs from nonimportant ones, represent crucial life skills.

Q: *What is the most important factor in productivity?*

The most important factor is clearly our emotional state during the work situation. When we are feeling motivated, relaxed, determined, energized, calm, and confident, high productivity will naturally follow. Sustaining an Ideal Performance State during work is the most important factor in productivity.

Q: *Of all the strategies available for toughening, which is the most powerful?*

If I could choose only one training method for accelerating life toughening, it would be physical exercise. Exercise is a wonderful vehicle for administering controlled doses of stress and recovery. Increases in physical toughness automatically lead to gains in mental and emotional toughness as well.

Q: *How should we view stress in our lives?*

Stress is life. Without stress we quickly become helpless and weak. Stress is essential for growth, happiness, and health. Freedom from stress simply breeds dysfunction and illness. To get the most out of life, we must become *stress seekers*.

Q: *What does "making waves" mean?*

Making waves means making cycles—cycles of stress and recovery. The more the better. The higher the better. We need to oscillate, move, change. We need to make waves, lots of waves—mental, physical, emotional.

The opposite of wave making is linearity. The more linear we become in our lives, the less productive, less happy, and less healthy we will be. All stress without recovery becomes linear, and all recovery without stress becomes linear. To get the most out of life we must pulsate, oscillate, and vibrate.

SUMMARY

Life is clearly a battle. The compelling message of life today is that it's tough—real tough—and getting tougher all the time. Like elite soldiers, we must train to be strong enough to fight courageously with passion and fervent optimism. Our battle is for life—for fulfillment, balance, and personal happiness. The enemy is ignorance, defensiveness, weakness, and fear. We must summon all the forces from within and move bravely to the front lines.

To get tougher in life, we must forge beyond our comfort zone. We must stretch to new limits, fall back and regroup, and then again march courageously forward into new and perhaps strange and frightening territories.

Every precious day of life becomes another opportunity to grow in flexibility, responsiveness, strength, and resiliency. And when the storms of life descend, as they most certainly will, our toughness is there to sustain and protect us. In fact, we can emerge from battle even tougher, more balanced, more skillful, more hopeful. And our rewards for victory are immense: maximum happiness, productivity, and health.

It is my sincerest hope that this book will help you in your quest for personal victory. Get tougher and tougher, get even tougher, toughen yourself again and again, and then do it some more. Never surrender, certainly not to the petty frustrations of daily living, not to the greatest crisis of your life, not even to time itself. Never, never surrender!

GLOSSARY

ACTH The adrenocorticotropic hormone that stimulates the outer layer of the adrenal gland.

adaptation threshold The maximum amount of physical or emotional stress an individual can handle.

adaptation Internal changes that reflect the toughening process. Most adaptations are easily measured in physical toughening (bench pressing twice the weight, for example, or increased muscle size). However, adaptations are no less real in emotional or mental toughening, although the measuring techniques must be more sophisticated.

adrenal glands Endocrine, or ductless, glands that are located on top of each kidney. They have two components. The first is the adrenal medulla, which produces and releases the hormones epinephrine and norepinephrine. The second is the adrenal cortex, which produces the hormone cortisol.

aerobic   In the presence of oxygen.

aerobic exercise   Endurance-type exercise of moderate intensity (65 to 80 percent of estimated maximum heart rate is commonly used as the range of aerobic intensity). Usually defined in terms of continuous activity of the large muscles.

anaerobic   In the absence of oxygen.

anaerobic exercise   Speed or power-type exercise of moderate to high intensity. The metabolic demands of the exercise cannot be met entirely by oxygen supplied from respiration.

ATP   Adenosine triphosphate, the nucleotide that supplies energy. Found in the muscles.

autonomic   Acting or happening involuntarily. An important part of our nervous system operates autonomically.

B cell   A type of immune cell capable of producing antibodies.

carbohydrate   A food substance including various sugars and starches. Found in fruits, vegetables, grains, rice, and potatoes. Carbohydrates convert to glucose in the blood and to glycogen in the muscles and liver.

catecholamines   A class of compounds that includes the two hormones epinephrine and norepinephrine, which are produced by the adrenal medulla.

chronic   Extending over a prolonged period of time.

circadian rhythms   Biological rhythms that rise and fall every 24 hours.

cortex   Outer layer. The adrenal cortex is the outer layer of the adrenal gland.

cortisol   One of the primary hormones produced and released by the adrenal cortex. Cortisol appears to play a central role in negative arousal. Often associated with feelings of fear, tension, and pressure, cortisol is one of the principal corticosteroid hormones responsible for the suppression of the immune system.

discomfort　A signal to pay attention. See **pain**.

Electrical Skin Resistance (ESR)　A measure of stress resulting from the electrical resistance of the skin.

electrocardiogram (EKG)　The heartbeat rendered electronically as a series of dips and spikes on a monitor for instant readout, or on paper when a record is desired.

electroencephalogram (EEG)　A recording of the brain's electrical activity.

electromyogram (EMG)　The recording of the electrical activity of a muscle.

endocrine gland　A gland that produces hormones and releases them directly into the bloodstream. Also called ductless gland.

endorphin　One of the neuropeptides, this morphinelike brain hormone stimulates the immune cells. Endorphin can produce a sense of well-being and mask pain.

epinephrine　One of the principal hormones of the adrenal medulla, commonly called adrenaline. Epinephrine plays a central role in positive arousal and is associated with increased feelings of energy, alertness, and concentration.

glucocorticoids　A group of natural steroid hormones released by the adrenal gland.

glucose　A simple sugar transported by the blood.

glycogen　A stored form of carbohydrate found principally in the muscles and liver.

health A state characterized by action, movement, oscillation, and pulsation. The goal of health-seekers should be physical and emotional nonlinearity, in which the dynamic interactions of stress and recovery are in balance. This balance brings psychological and physical harmony and synchrony, more commonly called health.

healthiness Healthiness is the direct consequence of regular, repeated cycles of balanced stress and recovery.

hypothalamus An area of the brain believed to be responsible for controlling and releasing a variety of pituitary hormones. Believed to be important in the regulation of emotion.

Ideal Performance State (IPS) The most effective mental, emotional, and physical state for performing at one's highest capability. The IPS is characterized by a specific constellation of positive feelings and emotions—calmness, relaxation, confidence, joy, and a sense of fun and fulfillment.

interval training Exercise program that alternates fast-slow or hard-easy work. Variable work output as opposed to steady-state output.

IPS control The ability to put oneself into the Ideal Performance State whenever desired in order to function at one's highest level. This priceless skill is acquired through Toughness Training.

leukocyte An immune cell that increases as much as four times over resting levels during exercise. The rate of increase depends on the duration and intensity of the exercise and the fitness level of the exerciser.

limbic system The limbic system of the brain is thought to be the control center of emotion.

linearity Habits or routines that are rigid and unvarying from a straight line, the opposite of the oscillating cycles of stress and recovery that characterize action, movement, and toughening.

linear recovery When energy recovery exceeds stress, the unbalanced condition causes weakening rather than toughening.

linear stress This weakening condition occurs when energy expenditure is not balanced by recovery.

lymphocyte A type of immune cell that increases in number during and immediately following exercise. However, the numbers of lymphocyte cells decrease below resting levels following long-distance running.

maintenance stress Exposure to normal stress and recovery that merely maintains current toughness levels.

negative arousal Pituitary-adrenal-cortical stimulation resulting from the perception of threat and experienced as unpleasant.

negative emotions Feelings that are experienced as unpleasant such as guilt, anger, or fear. Referred to in the context of psychological pain, negative emotions are critical barometers of excessive stress. Compare to **positive emotions**.

negative stress Energy expenditure accompanied by physical or emotional pain. This is the kind of stress most likely to weaken you. Compare to **positive stress**.

negative stressors Situations or stimuli that cause physical or emotional pain.

neuropeptides Small proteinlike chemicals produced by the brain cells. Neuropeptides have powerful mood-stimulating effects and provide the chemical basis of emotion. At least one of them, endorphin, also acts as a pain reliever. High concentrations of neuropeptides are found in the limbic system of the brain.

nonlinearity The dynamic interactions of stress and recovery that, when balanced, bring psychological and physical harmony and synchrony, better known as **health**.

"no pain, no gain" This is probably the most dangerous concept in physical training. A more realistic idea is "Pain prevents gain." See Chapter 2.

norepinephrine Often called noradrenaline, this is one of the principal hormones secreted by the adrenal medulla. Norepine-phrine plays a central role in positive arousal and is also a chemical transmitter substance at nerve endings. Classified as a catechola-mine.

one repetition maximum (1 RM) The maximum weight a person can lift one time.

overload To stress beyond normal limits.

overload principle Strength gains occur only when muscles are stressed (loaded) beyond the point to which they are normally stressed. See **overstress**.

overstress The overload principle must be applied with care. If the level of resistance is too great for current capacities, the muscles being overstressed may actually lose rather than gain strength. Overstressing also involves high risks of injury.

overtraining Results when more stress than recovery is present over an extended period of time. Flexibility, responsiveness, strength, and resiliency all decline in overtraining, resulting in weakening.

pain Physical or emotional pain is a signal to stop. "No pain, no gain" is a dangerous idea. See Chapter 2.

pituitary-adrenal-cortical arousal The primary stress response linked to cortisol release. Referred to in the context of **negative arousal**.

positive arousal SNS-adrenal-medullary stimulation resulting from the perception of challenge and experienced as pleasant.

positive emotions Feelings that are experienced as pleasant such as joy, love, pleasure, laughter, and confidence. Compare to **negative emotions**.

positive energy Energy generated from positive emotions. High positive energy, a critical factor in peak performance, results when cycles of stress and recovery are continuously balanced.

positive stress Energy expenditure without physical or emotional pain is positive stress, the kind most likely to toughen you. Compare to **negative stress**.

protection Excessive protection from stress breeds linearity, which in any form eventually becomes dysfunctional and unhealthy.

range of coping The volume of stress an individual is capable of handling without beginning to break down.

reactivity The ability to increase catecholamine levels quickly and sensitively in response to stress.

recovery Anything that causes energy to be recaptured—rest, relaxation, sleep, meditation, food, drink, diversion, and the like. Recovery is a biochemical event. Compare to **stress**.

SNS-adrenal-medullary arousal The primary stress response linked to catecholamine release. Referred to in the context of **positive arousal**.

stress Anything that causes energy to be expended. Compare to **recovery**. All forms of stress are biochemical events. Mental and emotional stress is just as real as physical stress, because energy expenditure occurs physically, mentally, and emotionally.

stress management The art and science of balancing the nearly endless symphony of pulsating stress/recovery clocks running inside all human beings.

stressors The specific causes of energy expenditure. Examples of physical stressors: walking, running, swimming, and, in fact, any physical movement at all. Emotional stressors: losing an order, making a presentation, feeling conflicting demands. Mental stressors: studying new material, solving difficult math problems, memorizing.

sympathetic nervous system   One of two major divisions of the **autonomic** nervous system.

tough   Characteristic of a vibrant state of being that's fluctuating, not stationary; dynamic, not static. Its measure is flexibility, responsiveness, strength, and resiliency under stress.

toughen   To toughen is to follow a course of training that makes the trainee more flexible, responsive, strong, and resilient, either emotionally or physically, in response to stress. Compare to **weaken**.

Toughness Training   May be either physical, mental, or emotional. Exposes an individual to positive challenges of sufficient intensity to cause adaptation to a higher level of stress. Toughening results from the systematic and precise administration of cycles of energy expenditure (stress) alternating with properly balanced cycles of energy recovery (rest).

undertraining   Occurs when one indulges in more recovery than stress over an extended period of time. This absence of challenge weakens the overly rested individual in every sphere—physical, emotional, and mental—in which the excessive rest occurs.

weaken   To become less flexible, responsive, strong, and resilient, either physically or emotionally, in response to stress. Compare to **toughen**.

weakened   Weakened people respond to stress in rigid, defensive, nonadaptive ways, particularly in nonsport situations. Their often slow and indecisive responses usually lack energy and force. Weakened individuals also show a marked inability to recover quickly from episodes of stress.

SELECTED REFERENCES

The publications included in this section are provided as resource material for readers who wish to explore topics in greater depth.

Abbreviations
JAMA   Journal of the American Medical Association
JAP   Journal of Applied Physiology
JCEPP   Journal of Clinical Experimental Pharmacology and Physiology
NEJM   New England Journal of Medicine

ADER, R. *Psychoneuroimmunology,* vol. 2. New York: Academic Press, 1981.

ALBANES, D., BLAIR, A., AND TAYLOR, P. R. "Physical Activity and Risk of Cancer in the NHANES I Population." *American Journal of Public Health* 79, 744–50, 1989.

ATHA, J. "Strengthening Muscle." *Exercise and Sport Science Reviews* 9, 1–70, 1981.

BAILEY, C. *The Fit or Fat Woman.* Boston: Houghton Mifflin, 1989. ————. *The New Fit or Fat.* Boston: Houghton Mifflin, 1991.

BALLARD-BARBASH, R., SCHATZKIN, A., ALBANES, D., SCHIFFMAN, M. H., KREGOR, B. E., KENNEL, W. B., ANDERSON, K. M., AND HELSEL, W. E. "Physical Activity and Risk of Large Bowel Cancer in the Framingham Study." *Cancer Research* 50, 3610–13, 1990.

BARCHAS, J. D., AND FREEDMAN, D. X. "Brain Amines: Response to Physiological Stress." *Biochem. Pharmacol.* 12, 1232–35, 1963.

BEECHER, H. "The Powerful Placebo." *JAMA* 159, 1602–5, 1955.

BLAYLOCK, J. E., WEIGENT, D. A. "Expression of Growth Hormone by Lymphocytes." *International Review of Immunology* 4, 195–213.

BORTZ, W. M., ET AL. "Catecholamines, Dopamine and Endorphin Levels During Extreme Exercise." *NEJM* 305, NO8, 1981.

BRAHMI, Z., THOMAS, J. E., PARK, M., AND DOWDESWELL, I. R. G. "The Effect of Acute Exercise on Natural Killer-Cell Activity of Trained and Sedentary Human Subjects." *Journal of Clinical Immunology* 5, 321–28, 1985.

BROOKS, S. M. E., NEVILL, L., MELEAGROS, H., LAKOMY, K. A., BLOOM, S. R., AND WILLIAMS, C. "The Hormonal Responses to Repetitive Brief Maximal Exercise in Humans." *European Journal of Physiologies* 60, 144–48, 1990.

BRYAN, R. M. "Cerebral Blood Flow and Energy Metabolism During Stress." *American Journal of Physiology* 259, H 269–80, 1990.

BRYNTESON, P., AND SINNING, W. E. "The Effects of Training Frequencies on the Retention of Cardiovascular Fitness." *Medicine and Science in Sports* 5, 29–30, 1974.

CLARK, D. H. "Adaptations in Strength and Muscular Endurance Resulting from Exercise." *Exercise and Sport Science Reviews* 1, 73–100, 1973.

COBB, S. "Social Support as a Moderator of Life Stress." *Psychosomatic Medicine* 38, 300–10, 1976.

COOPER, K. *The Aerobics Program for Total Well-Being.* New York: Bantam, 1982.

CORNELIUS, U. L. "Flexibility: The Effective Way." *National Strength and Conditioning Association Journal* 7, 62–65, 1985.

COSTILL, D. L., COYLE, E. F., FINK, W. F., LESMES, G. R., AND WITZMANN, F. A. "Adaptations in Skeletal Muscle Following Strength Training." *JAP* 46, 96–98, 1979.

COWLES, W. N. "Fatigue as a Contributory Cause of Pneumonia." *Boston Medical and Surgery Journal* 179, 555, 1918.

DARDIK, I. "Cardiocybernetics: Relaxation Through Exercise." *Advances* 3, 56–59, 1986.

DEVRIS, H. A. *Physiology of Exercise for Physical Education and Athletes.* Dubuque: Brown, 1980.

DIENSTBIER, R. "Arousal and Physiological Toughness: Implications for Mental and Physical Health." *Psych. Review* 96:1, 84–100, 1989.

————. "Behavioral Correlates of Sympathoadrenal Reactivity: The Toughness Model." *Medicine and Science in Sport and Exercise* 23:7, 846–52, 1991.

————, ET AL. "Catecholamine Training Effects from Exercise Programs: A Bridge to Exercise-Temperament Relationships." *Motivation and Emotion* 2, 297–318, 1987.

DORIAN, B., AND GARFINKEL, P. E. "Stress, Immunity and Illness: A Review." *Psychological Medicine* 17, 393–407, 1987.

DUSTMAN, R. E., ET AL. "Age and Fitness Effects on EEG, ERPs, Visual Sensitivity, and Cognition." *Neurobiology of Aging,* 11, 193–200, 1990.

EKMAN, P., AND OSTER, H. *The Facial Action Coding System.* Palo Alto: Consulting Psychologists Press, 1979.

EVANS, F. "Unravelling Placebo Effects: Expectations and the Placebo Response." *Advances* 1:3, 11–20, 1984.

FLECK, S. J., AND KRAEMER, W. J. *Designing Resistance Training Programs.* Champaign: Human Kinetics, 1987.

FOX, E. L., AND MATHEWS, D. K. *Interval Training.* Philadelphia: Saunders, 1974.

FRIEDRICH, J. *The Pre-Menstrual Solution.* San Jose: Arrow Press, 1987.

GARFINKEL, P. *In a Man's World.* New York: New American Library, 1985.

GIMINEZ, M., MOHAN-KUMAR, T., HUMBERT, T., DE TALANCE, J. C., TEBOUL, N., AND BELENGUER, F. J. A. "Training and Leucocyte, Lymphocyte and Platelet Response to Dynamic Exercise." *Journal of Sports Medicine* 27, 172–77, 1987.

GUILLEMIN, R., COHN, M., AND MELNECHUK, T. *Neural Modulation of Immunity.* New York: Raven Press, 1985. Pp. 29–40.

HADDEN, J. W., MASEK, K., AND NISTILO, G. *Interactions Among Central Nervous, Neuroendocrine and Immune Systems.* Rome/Milan: Pythagora Press, 1989.

HALL, N. R. S., AND GOLDSTEIN, A. L. "Thinking Well: The Chemical Links Between Emotions and Health." *The Sciences,* 34–41, 1986.

HALL, N. R. S., AND KVARNES, R. *International Perspectives on Self-Regulation and Healing.* Ed. J. Carlsen and R. Seifert. New York: Plenum, 1991. Pp. 183–95.

HILL, S., GOETZ, F. C., FOX, H. M., MURAWSKI, B. J., KRAKAUER, L. J., REIFENSTEIN, R. W., GRAY, S. J., REDDY, W. J., HEDBERG, S. E., ST. MARC, J. R., AND THORN, G. W. "Studies on Adrenocortical and Psychological Response to Stress in Man." *American Medical Association Archives of Internal Medicine* 97, 269–90, 1956.

IRWIN, M., DANIELS, M., BLOOM, E., SMITH, T., AND WEINER, H. "Life Events, Depression Systems, and Immune Function." *American Journal of Psychiatry* 144, 437–40, 1987.

JENKINS, D., ET AL. "Nibbling Versus Gorging: Metabolic Advantages of Increased Meal Frequency." *NEJM* 321:14, 929–35, 1989.

KAUFMANN, E. "The New Rhythm of Fitness." *American Health*, December 1989.

KJAER, M., CHRISTENSEN, N. J., SONNE, B., RICHTER, E. A., AND GALBO, H. "The Effect of Exercise on Epinephrine Turnover in Trained and Untrained Man." *JAP* 59, 1061–67, 1985.

KJAER, M., AND GALBO, H. "The Effect of Physical Training on the Capacity to Secrete Epinephrine." *JAP* 64, 11–16, 1988.

KLOPFER, B. "Psychological Variables in Human Cancer." *Journal of Projective Techniques* 21, 337–38, 1957.

KRAEMER, W. J., ET AL. "Hypothalamic-Pituitary-Adrenal Responses to Short-Duration High Intensity Cycle Exercise." *JAP* 68, 161–66, 1989.

———. "Effects of High Intensity Cycle Exercise on Sympathoadrenal-medullary Response Patterns." *JAP* 70, 8–14, 1991.

KRIGERS, H., AND KEITZER, H. A. "Overtraining in Elite Athletes." *Sports Medicine* 6, 79–92, 1988.

LE DOUX, J. E. "Cognitive-Emotional Interactions in the Brain." *Cognition and Emotion* 3, 267, 1989.

LLOYD, D., AND ROSSI, E., eds. *High Frequency Biological Rhythms: Functions of the Ultradians.* New York: Springer-Verlag, 1992.

LOEHR, J. *Mental Toughness Training for Sports.* New York: Penguin, 1986.

————, AND MCLAUGHLIN, P. *Mentally Tough.* New York: Evans, 1986.

MACKINNON, L. *Exercise and Immunology.* Champaign: Human Kinetics, 1982.

MAFFULLI, N. "Intensive Training in Young Athletes." *Sports Medicine* 9, 229–43, 1990.

MANYANDE, M., CHAYEN, S., PRIYAKUMAR, P., CHRISTOPHER, C., SMITH, T., HAYES, M., HIGGINS, D., KEE, S., PHILLIPS, S., AND SALMON, P. "Anxiety and Endrocrine Responses to Surgery: Paradoxical Effects of Preoperative Relaxation Training." *Psychosomatic Medicine* 54, 275–87, 1992.

MARKOFF, R. A., RYAN, P., AND YOUNG, T. "Endorphins and Mood Changes in Long Distance Running." *Med. Sci. Sports Exerc.* 14:1, 11–15, 1992.

MARTENS, R. *Joy and Sadness in Children's Sports.* Champaign: Human Kinetics, 1978.

MASLOW, A. *Toward a Psychology of Being,* vol. 3. New York: Van Nostrand Reinhold, 1968.

MCCARTHY, D., AND DALE, M. "The Leucocytosis of Exercise: A Review and Model." *Sports Medicine* 6, 333–60, 1988.

MCMURRAY, R. G., FORSYTHE, W. A., MAR, M. H., AND HARDY, C. J. "Exercise Intensity–Related Responses in B-endorphin and Catecholamines." *Med. Sci. Sports Exerc.* 19:6, 570–74, 1987.

MELNECHUK, T. "Emotions, Brain, Immunity, and Health: A Review." In Clynes and Panksepp, eds., *Emotions and Psychopathology.* New York: Plenum, 1988.

NIEMAN, D. C., BERK, L. S., ET AL. "Effects of Long-Endurance Running on Immune Systems Parameters and Lymphocyte Functions in Experienced Marathoners." *International Journal of Sports Medicine* 10, 317–23.

NIEMAN, D. C., JOHANSSEN, L. M., LEE, J. W., AND ARABATYIS, K. "Infectious Episodes in Runners Before and After the Los Angeles Marathon." *Journal of Sports Medicine and Physical Fitness* 30, 316–28, 1990.

OOMUR, Y. *Emotions: Neural and Chemical Control.* Tokyo: Japan Scientific Societies Press, 1988.

OSHIDA, Y., YAMANOUCHI, K., HSYAMIZU, S., AND SATO, Y. "Effect of Acute Physical Exercise on Lymphocyte Subpopulations in Trained and Untrained Subjects." *International Journal of Sports Medicine* 9, 137–40, 1988.

PEARSALL, P. *Super-Immunity.* New York: McGraw-Hill, 1987.

PERT, C., RUFF, M., WEBER, R., AND HERKENHAM, M. "Neuropeptides and Their Receptors: A Psychosomatic Network." *Journal of Immunology* 135:2, 8205–45, 1985.

PESTELL, R. G., HURLEY, D. M., AND VANDONGEN, R. "Biochemical and Hormonal Changes During a 100 Km Ultramarathon." *Clin. Exp. Pharmacol. Physiology* 16, 353–61, 1989.

PETERS, E. M., AND BATEMAN, E. D. "Ultramarathon Running and Upper Respiratory Tract Infections." *South African Medical Journal* 64, 582–84, 1983.

PFEIFER, W. D. "Modification of Adrenal Tyrosine Hydroxylase Activity in Rats Following Manipulation in Infancy." In E. Usdin, Kvetnansky, and Kopin, eds., *Catecholamines and Stress*. Oxford, England: Pergamon (n.d.). Pp. 265–70.

RENOLD, A. E., QUIGLEY, T. B., KENARD, H. E., AND THORN, G. W. "Reaction of the Adrenal Cortex to Physical and Emotional Stress in College Oarsmen." *NEJM* 244, 754–58, 1951.

RESTAK, R. *The Brain*. New York: Bantam, 1984.

ROLLS, E. T. "Theory of Emotion, and Its Application to Understanding the Neural Basis of Emotion." In Y. Oomur, ed., *Emotions: Neural and Chemical Control*. Tokyo: Japan Scientific Societies Press, 1988. Pp. 325–44.

ROSSI, E. *The 20-Minute Break*. Los Angeles: Tarcher, 1991.

———. "The Wave Nature of Consciousness." *Psychological Perspectives* 24, 1–6, 1991.

RYAN, A. J., BROWN, R. L., FREDRICK, E. C., FALSETTI, H. L., AND BURKE, R. E. "Overtraining of Athletes: A Round Table." *Phys. Sportsmed.* 11, 93–110, 1983.

SALTIN, B., AND ROWELL, L. B. "Functional Adaptations to Physical Activity and Inactivity." *Federation Proceedings* 39, 1506–19, 1980.

SCHULTZ, H., AND LOVIE, P. *Ultradian Rhythms in Physiology and Behavior*. New York: Springer-Verlag, 1985.

SCHWARTZ, T. "Making Waves." *New York,* March 18, 1989, 31–39.

SCHWARZ, L., AND KINDERMANN, W. "Beta-endorphin Catecholamines and Cortisol During Exhaustive Endurance Exercise." *International Journal of Sports Medicine* 10, 324–28, 1989.

SHELLOCK, F. G., AND PRENTICE, W. E. "Warming Up and Stretching for Improved Physical Performance and Prevention of Sports Related Injuries." *Sports Medicine* 2, 267–77, 1985.

SIMONTON, C., MATTHEWS-SIMONTON, S., AND CREIGHTON, J. *Getting Well Again.* Los Angeles: Tarcher, 1978.

STALLSNECHT, B., ET AL. "Diminished Epinephrine Response to Hypoglycemia Despite Enlarged Adrenal Medulla in Trained Rats." *American Journal of Physiology* 259, R998–R1003, 1990.

STEIN, M. "Bereavement, Depression, Stress and Immunity." In R. Guillemin, M. Cohen, and T. Melnechuk, eds., *Neural Modulation of Immunity.* New York: Raven Press, 1985. Pp. 29–44.

STONE, M. H., ET AL. "Overtraining: A Review of the Signs, Symptoms and Possible Causes." *Journal of Appl. Sport Sci. Research* 5:1, 35–50, 1991.

URSIN, H., ET AL. "Conclusion: Sustained Activation and Disease." In H. Ursin and R. Murison, eds., *Biological and Psychological Basis of Psychosomatic Disease.* Oxford, England: Pergamon, 1983. Pp. 269–77.

WALTON, G. *Beyond Winning: The Timeless Wisdom of Great Philosopher Coaches.* Champaign: Human Kinetics, 1992.

WEISS, J. M., ET AL. "Effects of Chronic Exposure to Stressors on Avoidance-Escape Behavior and on Brain Norepinephrine." *Psychosomatic Medicine* 37, 522–34, 1975.

WILLIAMS, J. M., AND GETTY, D. "Effects of Levels of Exercise on Psychological Mood States, Physical Fitness and Plasma Beta-endorphin." *Percept. Mot. Skills* 63, 1099–1105, 1986.

INDEX